Your Guide to Breastfeeding

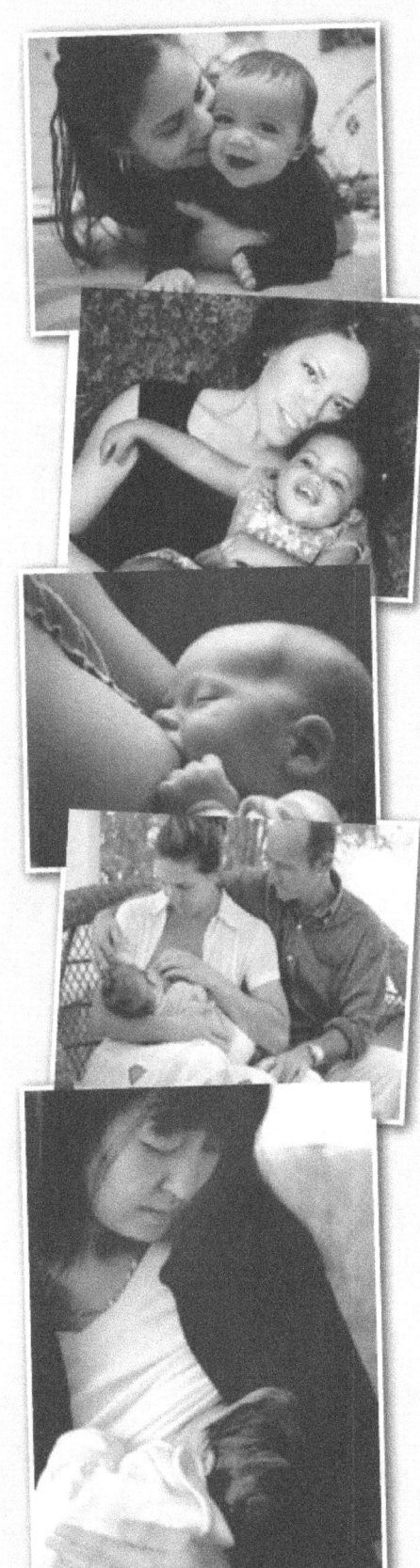

Introduction

The experience of breastfeeding is special for so many reasons, including:

- The joyful bonding with your baby
- The perfect nutrition only you can provide
- The cost savings
- The health benefits for both mother and baby

In fact, breast milk has disease-fighting antibodies that can help protect infants from several types of illnesses. And mothers who breastfeed have a lower risk of some health problems, including breast cancer and type 2 diabetes.

Keep in mind that breastfeeding is a learned skill. It requires patience and practice. For some women, the learning stages can be frustrating and uncomfortable. And some situations make breastfeeding even harder, such as babies born early or health problems in the mother. The good news is that it will get easier, and support for breastfeeding mothers is growing.

You are special because you can make the food that is uniquely perfect for your baby. Invest the time in yourself and your baby – for your health and for the bond that will last a lifetime.

The U.S. Department of Health and Human Services' Office on Women's Health (OWH) is raising awareness of the importance of breastfeeding to help mothers give their babies the best start possible in life. In addition to this guide, OWH offers online content at **http://www.womenshealth.gov/ breastfeeding** and provides the National Breastfeeding Helpline at 800-994-9662. *The Surgeon General's Call to Action to Support Breastfeeding* puts forth steps that family members, communities, clinicians, health care systems, and employers can take to make breastfeeding an easy choice for mothers. **Learn more at http://www.surgeongeneral.gov.** OWH also partners with the Health Resources and Services Administration's Maternal and Child Health Bureau to educate employers about the needs of breastfeeding mothers via *The Business Case for Breastfeeding*.

The Affordable Care Act (health care reform) helps pregnant women and breastfeeding mothers get the medical care and support they and their children need. Learn more at **http://www.healthcare.gov.**

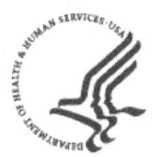

U.S. Department of Health and Human Services,
Office on Women's Health

January 2011

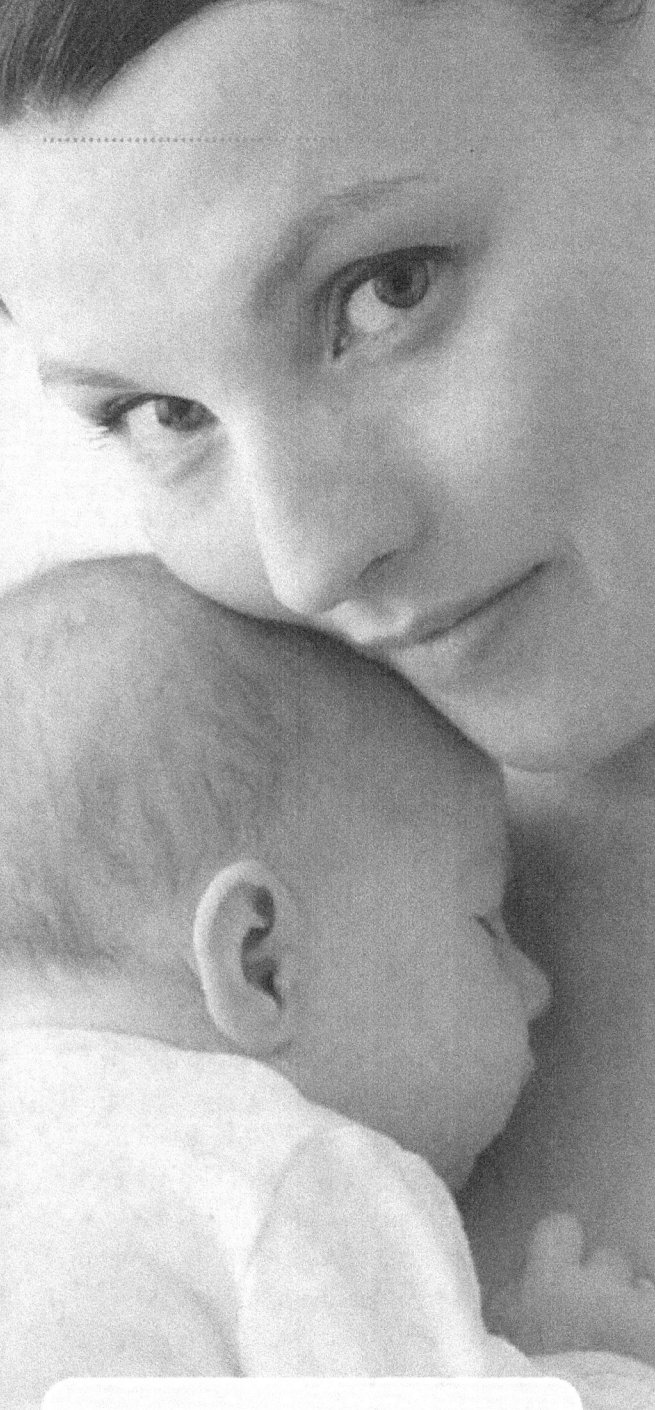

Contents

Tools you can use

Why Breastfeeding Is Important

Breastfeeding Protects Babies

1. **Early breast milk is liquid gold.**

    Known as liquid gold, colostrum (coh-LOSS-trum) is the thick yellow first breast milk that you make during pregnancy and just after birth. This milk is very rich in **nutrients** and **antibodies** to protect your baby. Although your baby only gets a small amount of colostrum at each feeding, it matches the amount his or her tiny stomach can hold. (See **page 17** to see just how small your newborn's tummy is!)

2. **Your breast milk changes as your baby grows.**

    Colostrum changes into what is called mature milk. By the third to fifth day after birth, this mature breast milk has just the right amount of fat, sugar, water, and protein to help your baby continue to grow. It is a thinner type of milk than colostrum, but it provides all of the nutrients and antibodies your baby needs.

3. **Breast milk is easier to digest.**

    For most babies – especially premature babies – breast milk is easier to digest than formula. The proteins in formula are made from cow's milk, and it takes time for babies' stomachs to adjust to digesting them.

4. **Breast milk fights disease.**

    The cells, hormones, and antibodies in breast milk protect babies from illness. This protection is unique; formula cannot match the chemical makeup of human breast milk. In fact, among formula-fed babies, ear infections and diarrhea are more common. Formula-fed babies also have higher risks of:

    *   Necrotizing (nek-roh-TEYE-zing) enterocolitis (en-TUR-oh-coh-lyt-iss), a disease that affects the gastrointestinal tract in pre-term infants.

    *   Lower respiratory infections

    *   Atopic dermatitis, a type of skin rash

    *   Asthma

    *   Obesity

    *   Type 1 and type 2 diabetes

    *   Childhood leukemia

Breastfeeding has also been shown to lower the risk of SIDS (sudden infant death syndrome).

Formula-feeding can raise health risks in babies, but there are rare cases in which formula may be a necessary alternative. Very rarely, babies are born unable to tolerate milk of any kind. These babies must have soy formula. Formula may also be needed if the mother has certain health conditions and she does not have access to donor breast milk. To learn more about rare breastfeeding restrictions in the mother, see **page 26**. To learn more about donor milk banks, see **page 32**.

Breastfeeding Glossary

Nutrients are any food substance that provides energy or helps build tissue.

Antibodies (AN-teye-bah-deez) are blood proteins made in response to germs or other foreign substances that enter the body. Antibodies help the body fight illness and disease by attaching to germs and marking them for destruction.

The **gastrointestinal system** is made up of the stomach, and the small and large intestines. It breaks down and absorbs food.

The **respiratory system** includes the nose, throat, voice box, windpipe, and lungs. Air is breathed in, delivering oxygen. Waste gas is removed from the lungs when you breathe out.

Mothers Benefit from Breastfeeding

1. **Ways that breastfeeding can make your life easier.**

    Breastfeeding may take a little more effort than formula feeding at first. But it can make life easier once you and your baby settle into a good routine. When you breastfeed, there are no bottles and nipples to sterilize. You do not have to buy, measure, and mix formula. And there are no bottles to warm in the middle of the night.

2. **Breastfeeding can save money.**

    Formula and feeding supplies can cost well over $1,500 each year, depending on how much your baby eats. Breastfed babies are also sick less often, which can lower health care costs.

3. **Breastfeeding can feel great.**

    Physical contact is important to newborns. It can help them feel more secure, warm, and comforted. Mothers can benefit from this closeness, as well. Breastfeeding requires a mother to take some quiet relaxed time to bond. The skin-to-skin contact can boost the mother's oxytocin (OKS-ee-TOH-suhn) levels. Oxytocin is a hormone that helps milk flow and can calm the mother.

4. **Breastfeeding can be good for the mother's health, too.**

    Breastfeeding is linked to a lower risk of these health problems in women:

    *   Type 2 diabetes
    *   Breast cancer
    *   Ovarian cancer
    *   Postpartum depression

    Experts are still looking at the effects of breastfeeding on osteoporosis and weight loss after birth. Many studies have reported greater weight loss for breastfeeding mothers than for those who don't. But more research is needed to understand if a strong link exists.

Breastfeeding During an Emergency

When an emergency occurs, breastfeeding can save lives:

*   Breastfeeding protects babies from the risks of a contaminated water supply.
*   Breastfeeding can help protect against respiratory illnesses and diarrhea. These diseases can be fatal in populations displaced by disaster.
*   Breast milk is the right temperature for babies and helps to prevent hypothermia when the body temperature drops too low.
*   Breast milk is readily available without needing other supplies.

5. **Nursing mothers miss less work.**

    Breastfeeding mothers miss fewer days from work because their infants are sick less often.

Breastfeeding Benefits Society

The nation benefits overall when mothers breastfeed. Recent research shows that if 90 percent of families breastfed exclusively for 6 months, nearly 1,000 deaths among infants could be prevented. The United States would also save $13 billion per year – medical care costs are lower for fully breastfed infants than for never-breastfed infants. Breastfed infants typically need fewer sick care visits, prescriptions, and hospitalizations.

Breastfeeding also contributes to a more productive workforce because mothers miss less work to care for sick infants. Employer medical costs are also lower.

Breastfeeding is also better for the environment. There is less trash and plastic waste compared to that produced by formula cans and bottle supplies.

Finding Support and Information

While breastfeeding is natural, you still may need some advice. There are many sources of support available for breastfeeding mothers. You can seek help from different types of health professionals, organizations, and members of your own family. Under the Affordable Care Act (health care reform), more and more women will have access to breastfeeding support without any out-of-pocket costs. And don't forget, friends who have successfully breastfed can be a great source of information and encouragement!

Health Professionals Who Help with Breastfeeding

Pediatricians, obstetricians, and certified nurse-midwives can help you with breastfeeding. Other special breastfeeding professionals include:

- **International Board Certified Lactation Consultant (IBCLC).** Lactation consultants are credentialed breastfeeding professionals with the highest level of knowledge and skill in breastfeeding support. IBCLCs are experienced in helping mothers to breastfeed comfortably by helping with positioning, latch, and a wide range of breastfeeding concerns. Many IBCLCs are also nurses, doctors, speech therapists, dietitians, or other kinds of health professionals. Ask your hospital or birthing center for the name of a lactation consultant who can help you. Or, you can go to http://www.ilca.org to find an IBCLC in your area.

- **Breastfeeding Peer Counselor or Educator.** A breastfeeding counselor can teach others about the benefits of breastfeeding and help women with basic breastfeeding challenges and questions. A "peer" means a person has breastfed her own baby and is available to help other mothers. Some breastfeeding educators have letters after their names like CLC (Certified Lactation Counselor) or CBE (Certified Breastfeeding Educator).

Educators have special breastfeeding training but not as much as IBCLCs. These professionals still can be quite helpful.

- **Doula (DOO-la).** A doula is professionally trained and experienced in giving social support to birthing families during pregnancy, labor, and birth and at home during the first few days or weeks after birth. Doulas who are trained in breastfeeding can help you be more successful with breastfeeding after birth.

Mother-to-Mother Support

Other breastfeeding mothers can be a great source of support. Mothers can share tips and offer one another encouragement. There are many ways you can connect with other breastfeeding mothers:

- Ask your health care provider or hospital staff to recommend a support group.

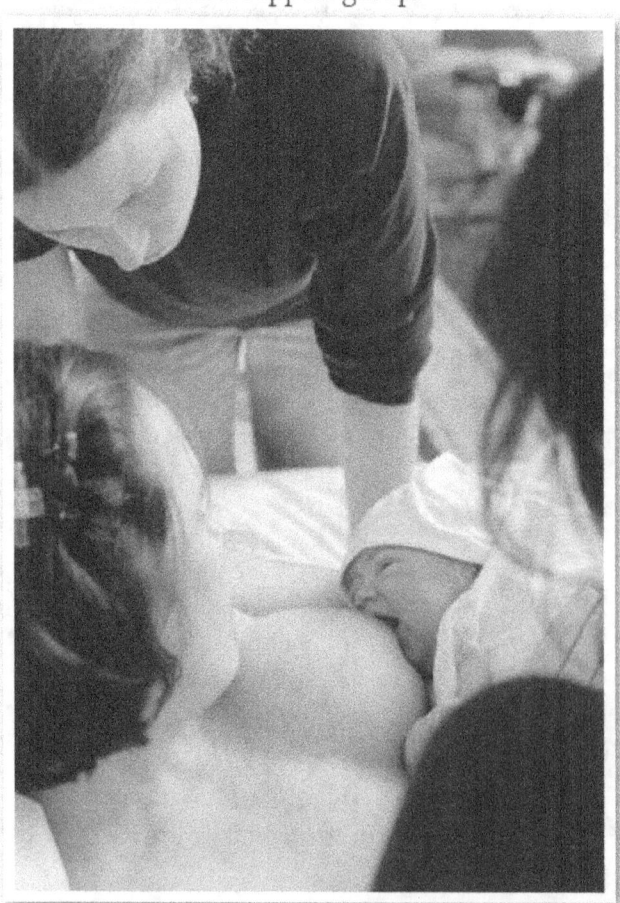

- Search your phone book or the Internet for a breastfeeding center near you. These centers may offer support groups.
- Find a local La Leche League support group by visiting the organization's website at http://www.llli.org/.
- Search the Internet for breastfeeding message boards and chats. (These resources can be great for sharing tips, but do not rely on websites for medical advice – talk to your health care provider.)

WIC Program

Food, nutrition counseling, and access to health services are provided to low-income women, infants, and children under the Special Supplemental Nutrition Program for Women, Infants, and Children. This program is popularly known as WIC (Women, Infants, and Children). Breastfeeding mothers supported by WIC may receive educational materials, peer counselor support, an enhanced food package, breast pumps, and other supplies.

Breastfeeding mothers are also eligible to participate in WIC longer than non-breastfeeding mothers. To find contact information for your local WIC program, visit http://www.fns.usda.gov/wic/Breastfeeding/breastfeedingmainpage.htm or call the national office at 703-305-2746.

Learn more about breastfeeding basics and find other online resources at http://www.womenshealth.gov/breastfeeding.

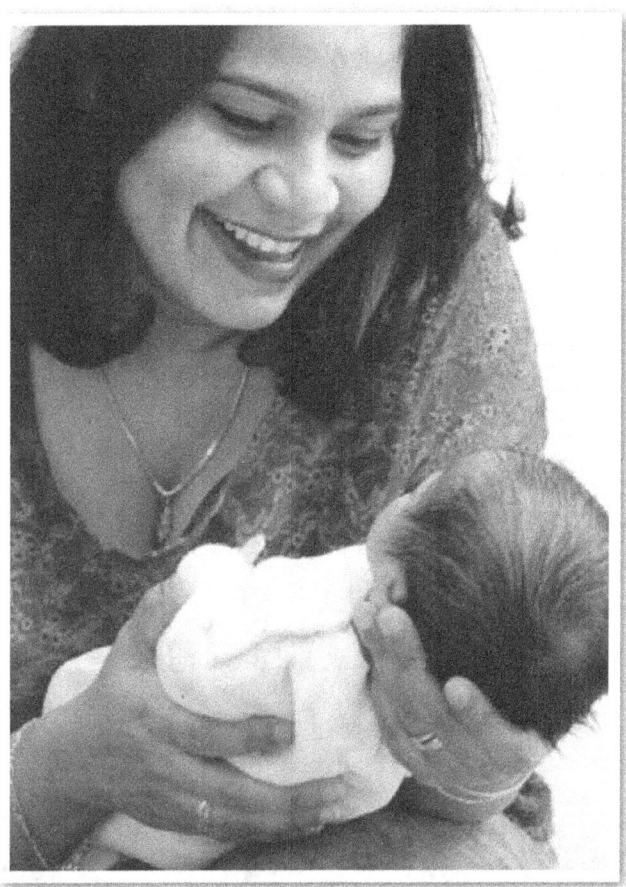

The National Breastfeeding Helpline

The National Breastfeeding Helpline from the Office on Women's Health has trained breastfeeding peer counselors to provide support by phone. The counselors can help answer common breastfeeding questions. They can also help you decide if you need to see a doctor or lactation consultant. The Helpline is available for all breastfeeding mothers, partners, prospective parents, family members, and health professionals seeking to learn more about breastfeeding. The Helpline is open from Monday through Friday, from 9 a.m. to 6 p.m., EST. If you call after hours, you will be able to leave a message, and a breastfeeding peer counselor will return your call on the next business day. Help is available in English or Spanish.

Call 800-994-9662 for Support!

How Breast Milk Is Made

Knowing how the breast works to produce milk can help you understand the breastfeeding process. The breast itself is a gland that is made up of several parts, including:

- **Glandular tissue** – body tissue that makes and releases one or more substances for use in the body. Some glands make fluids that affect tissues or organs. Others make hormones or assist with blood production. In the breast, this tissue is involved in milk production.

- **Connective tissue** – a type of body tissue that supports other tissues and binds them together. This tissue provides support in the breast.

- **Blood** – fluid in the body made up of plasma, red and white blood cells, and platelets. Blood carries oxygen and nutrients to and waste materials away from all body tissues. In the breast, blood nourishes the breast tissue and provides nutrients needed for milk production.

- **Lymph** – the almost colorless fluid that travels through the lymphatic system and carries cells that help fight infection and disease. Lymph tissue in the breast helps remove waste.

- **Nerves** – cells that are the building blocks of the nervous system (the system that records and transmits information chemically and electrically within a person). Nerve tissue in the breast makes breasts sensitive to touch, allowing the baby's sucking to stimulate the let-down or milk-ejection reflex and milk production. (See **page 9** to learn how let-down works!)

- **Fatty tissue** – connective tissue that contains stored fat. It is also known as adipose tissue. Fatty tissue in the breast protects the breast from injury. Fatty tissue is what mostly affects the size of a woman's breast. Breast size does not have an effect on the amount of milk or the quality of milk a woman makes.

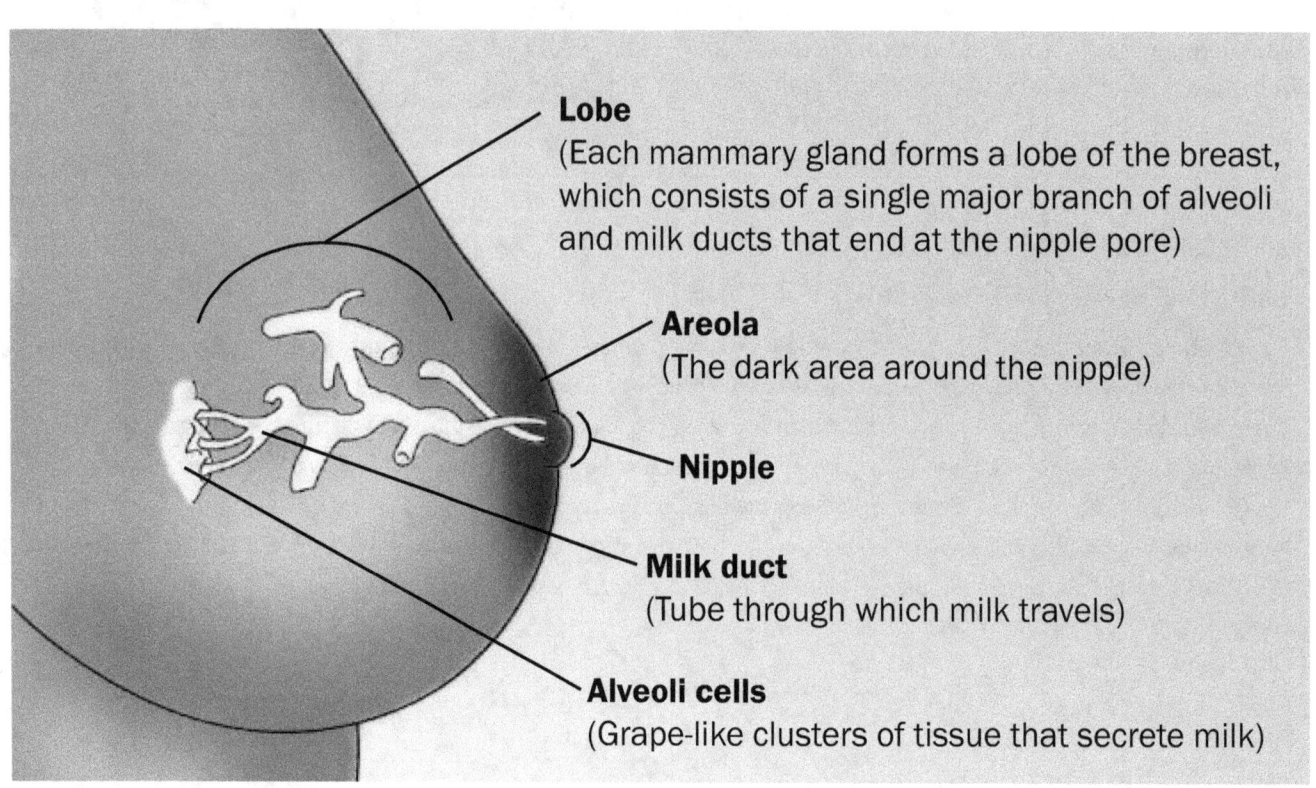

Lobe
(Each mammary gland forms a lobe of the breast, which consists of a single major branch of alveoli and milk ducts that end at the nipple pore)

Areola
(The dark area around the nipple)

Nipple

Milk duct
(Tube through which milk travels)

Alveoli cells
(Grape-like clusters of tissue that secrete milk)

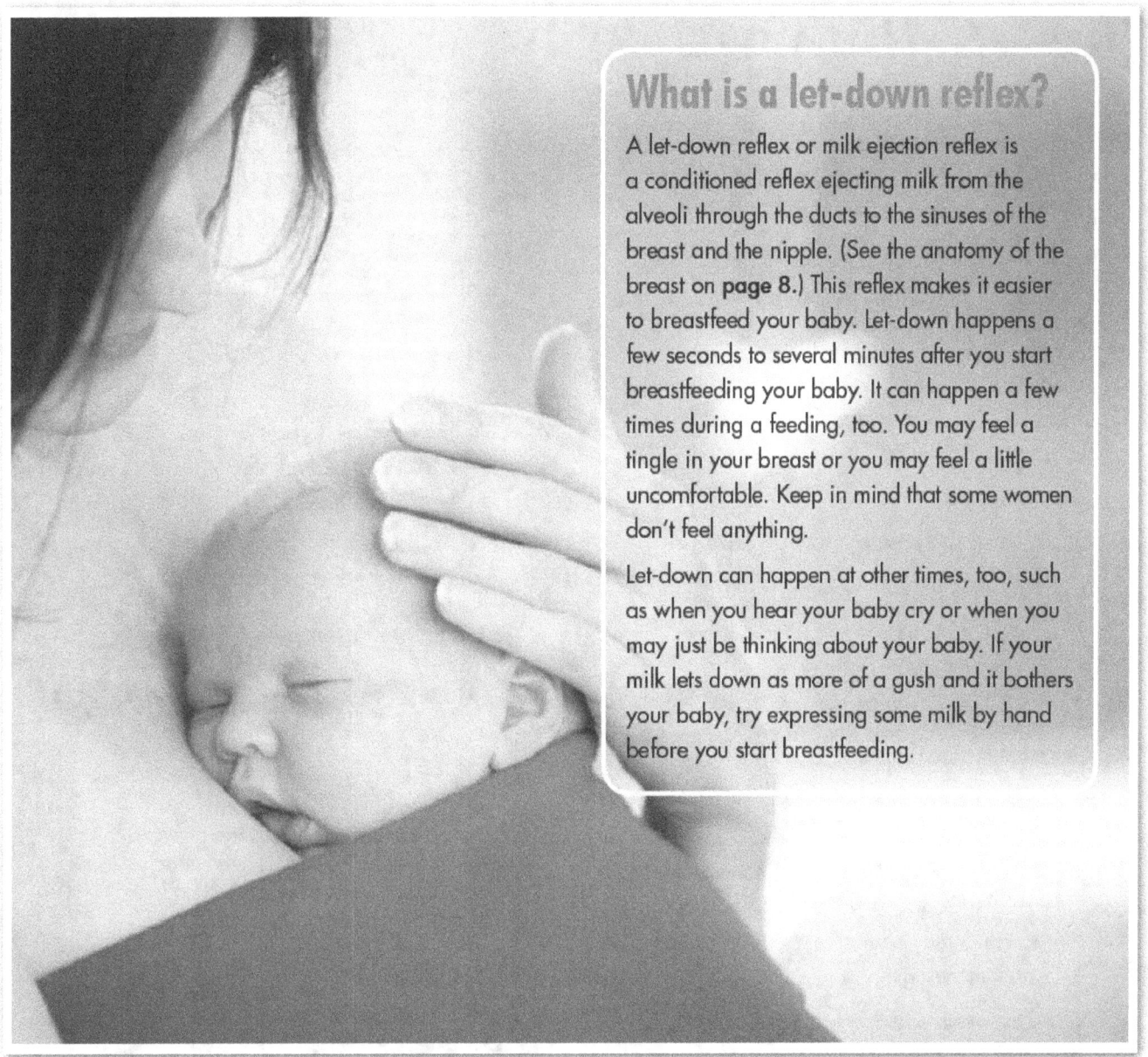

What is a let-down reflex?

A let-down reflex or milk ejection reflex is a conditioned reflex ejecting milk from the alveoli through the ducts to the sinuses of the breast and the nipple. (See the anatomy of the breast on **page 8**.) This reflex makes it easier to breastfeed your baby. Let-down happens a few seconds to several minutes after you start breastfeeding your baby. It can happen a few times during a feeding, too. You may feel a tingle in your breast or you may feel a little uncomfortable. Keep in mind that some women don't feel anything.

Let-down can happen at other times, too, such as when you hear your baby cry or when you may just be thinking about your baby. If your milk lets down as more of a gush and it bothers your baby, try expressing some milk by hand before you start breastfeeding.

Special cells inside your breasts make milk. These cells are called alveoli (al-VEE-uh-leye). When your breasts become fuller and tender during pregnancy, this is a sign that the alveoli are getting ready to work. Some women do not feel these changes in their breasts. Others may sense these changes after their baby is born.

The alveoli make milk in response to the hormone prolactin (proh-LAK-tin). Prolactin rises when the baby suckles. Another hormone, oxytocin (oks-ee-TOH-suhn), causes small muscles around the cells to contract and move the milk through a series of small tubes called milk ducts. This moving of the milk is called let-down reflex.

Oxytocin also causes the muscles of the uterus to contract during and after birth. This helps the uterus to get back to its original size. It also lessens any bleeding a woman may have after giving birth. The release of both prolactin and oxytocin may be responsible in part for a mother's intense feeling of needing to be with her baby.

Before You Give Birth

To prepare for breastfeeding, the most important thing you can do is have confidence in yourself. Committing to breastfeeding starts with the belief that you can do it!

Other steps you can take to prepare for breastfeeding:

1. Get good prenatal care, which can help you avoid early delivery. Babies born too early often need special care, which can make breastfeeding harder.

2. Take a breastfeeding class.

3. Ask your health care provider to recommend a lactation consultant. You can establish a relationship before the baby comes, or be ready if you need help after the baby is born.

4. Talk to your health care provider about your health. Discuss any breast surgery or injury you may have had. If you have depression or are taking medications, discuss treatment options that can work with breastfeeding.

5. Tell your health care provider that you would like to breastfeed your newborn baby as soon as possible after delivery. The sucking instinct is very strong within the first hour of life.

6. Talk to friends who have breastfed or consider joining a breastfeeding support group.

Talk to Fathers, Partners, and Other Family Members About How They Can Help

Breastfeeding is more than a way to feed a baby – it becomes a lifestyle. And fathers, partners, and other special support persons can be involved in the breastfeeding experience, too. Partners and family members can:

- Support the breastfeeding relationship by being kind and encouraging.

- Show their love and appreciation for all of the work that is put into breastfeeding.

- Be good listeners when a mother needs to talk through breastfeeding concerns.

- Make sure the mother has enough to drink and gets enough rest, help around the house, and take care of other children at home.

- Give emotional nourishment to the child through playing and cuddling.

Fathers, partners, and other people in the mother's support system can benefit from breastfeeding, too. Not only are there no bottles to prepare, but many people feel warmth, love, and relaxation just from sitting next to a mother and baby during breastfeeding.

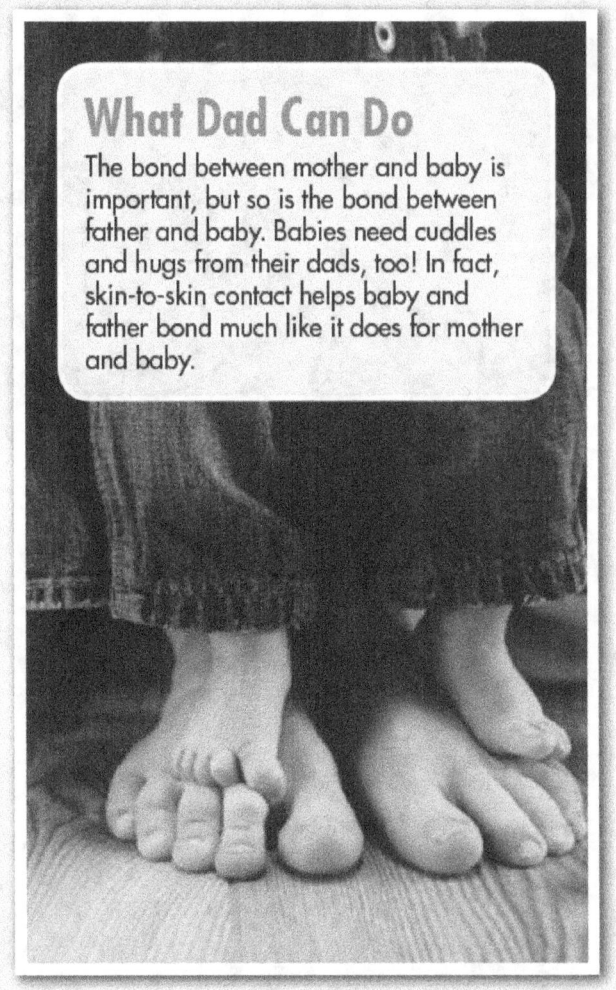

What Dad Can Do

The bond between mother and baby is important, but so is the bond between father and baby. Babies need cuddles and hugs from their dads, too! In fact, skin-to-skin contact helps baby and father bond much like it does for mother and baby.

Learning to Breastfeed

Breastfeeding is a process that takes time to master. Babies and mothers need to practice. Keep in mind that you make milk in response to your baby sucking at the breast. The more milk your baby removes from the breasts, the more milk you will make.

After you have the baby, these steps can help you get off to a great start:

- Breastfeed as soon as possible after birth.

- Ask for an on-site lactation consultant to come help you.

- Ask the staff not to give your baby other food or formula, unless it is medically necessary.

- Allow your baby to stay in your hospital room all day and night so that you can breastfeed often. Or, ask the nurses to bring your baby to you for feedings.

- Try to avoid giving your baby any pacifiers or artificial nipples so that he or she gets used to latching onto just your breast. (See **page 12** to learn about latching.)

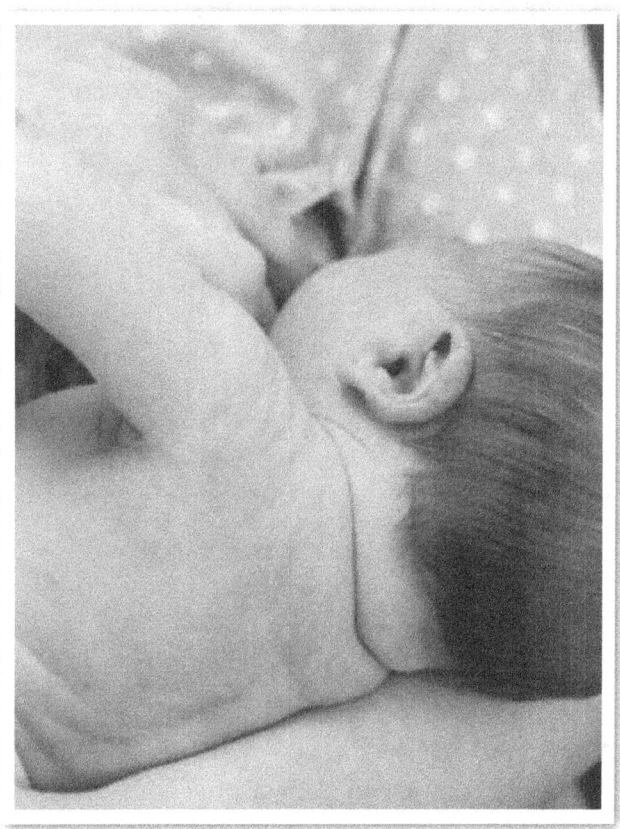

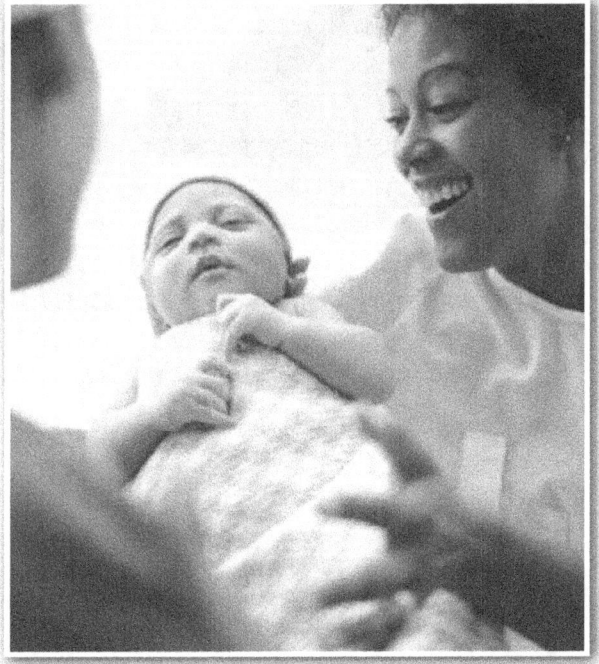

How often should I breastfeed?

Early and often! Breastfeed as soon as possible after birth, then breastfeed at least 8 to 12 times every 24 hours to make plenty of milk for your baby. This means that in the first few days after birth, your baby will likely need to breastfeed about every hour or two in the daytime and a couple of times at night. Healthy babies develop their own feeding schedules. Follow your baby's cues for when he or she is ready to eat.

How long should feedings be?

Feedings may be 15 to 20 minutes or longer per breast. But there is no set time. Your baby will let you know when he or she is finished. If you are worried that your baby is not eating enough, talk to your baby's doctor. See **page 45** for a feeding tracker if you would like to write down when your baby wants to eat.

Bringing Your Baby to the Breast

When awake, your baby will move his or her head back and forth, looking and feeling for the breast with his or her mouth and lips. The steps below can help you get your baby to "latch" on to the breast to start eating. Keep in mind that there is no one way to start breastfeeding. As long as the baby is latched on well, how you get there is up to you.

- Hold your baby, wearing only a diaper, against your bare chest. Hold the baby upright with his or her head under your chin. Your baby will be comfortable in that cozy valley between your breasts. You can ask your partner or a nurse to place a blanket across your baby's back and bring your bedcovers over you both. Your skin temperature will rise to warm your baby.

- Support his or her neck and shoulders with one hand and hips with the other. He or she may move in an effort to find your breast.

- Your baby's head should be tilted back slightly to make it easy to suck and swallow. With his or her head back and mouth open, the tongue is naturally down and ready for the breast to go on top of it.

- Allow your breast to hang naturally. When your baby feels it with his or her cheek, he or she may open his or her mouth wide and reach it up and over the nipple. You can also guide the baby to latch on as you see in these illustrations.

- At first, your baby's nose will be lined up opposite your nipple. As his or her chin presses into your breast, his or her wide open mouth will get a large mouthful of breast for a deep latch. Keep in mind that your baby can breathe at the breast. The nostrils flare to allow air in.

- Tilt your baby back, supporting your baby's head, upper back, and shoulders with the palm of your hand and pull your baby in close.

Some babies latch on right away, and for some it takes more time.

Getting your baby to latch:

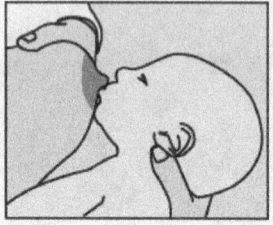

Tickle the baby's lips to encourage him or her to open wide.

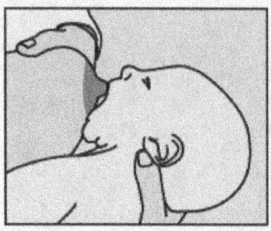

Pull your baby close so that the chin and lower jaw moves into your breast first.

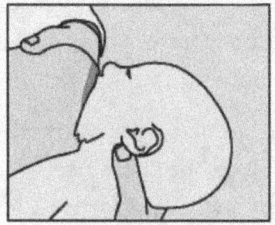

Watch the lower lip and aim it as far from the base of the nipple as possible, so the baby takes a large mouthful of breast.

When my son was born 4 years ago, we had a very difficult time breastfeeding because he wasn't latching correctly. He seemed almost lazy and disinterested in eating. In the first 2 weeks, he lost quite a bit of weight and appeared gaunt and fussy. Naturally, I was nearly frantic with worry. Luckily, I connected with an amazing lactation consultant. She put me on a rigorous, week-long regimen which consisted of nursing, then bottle feeding breast milk, then pumping every 3 hours. I was completely dedicated to the regimen, and when I met with her a week later, she was stunned by the results. My son had gained an entire pound, and she said he had developed a perfect latch. She called us the miracle mom and miracle baby! I was so proud of us. My determination paid off and I enjoyed breastfeeding for 7 months.
– Jill
Bridgewater, MA

Signs of a good latch

- The latch feels comfortable to you, without hurting or pinching. How it feels is more important than how it looks.

- Your baby's chest is against your body and he or she does not have to turn his or her head while drinking.

- You see little or no areola, depending on the size of your areola and the size of your baby's mouth. If areola is showing, you will see more above your baby's lip and less below.

- When your baby is positioned well, his or her mouth will be filled with breast.

- The tongue is cupped under the breast, although you might not see it.

- You hear or see your baby swallow. Some babies swallow so quietly, a pause in their breathing may be the only sign of swallowing.

- You see the baby's ears "wiggle" slightly.

- Your baby's lips turn out like fish lips, not in. You may not even be able to see the bottom lip.

- Your baby's chin touches your breast.

A Good Latch

A good latch is important for your baby to breastfeed effectively and for your comfort. During the early days of breastfeeding, it can take time and patience for your baby to latch on well.

Help with latch problems

Are you in pain? Many moms report that their breasts can be tender at first until both they and their baby find comfortable breastfeeding positions and a good latch. Once you have done this, breastfeeding should be comfortable. If it hurts, your baby may be sucking on only the nipple. Gently break your baby's suction to your breast by placing a clean finger in the corner of your baby's mouth and try again. Also, your nipple should not look flat or compressed when it comes out of your baby's mouth. It should look round and long, or the same shape as it was before the feeding.

Are you or your baby frustrated? Take a short break and hold your baby in an upright position. Try holding him or her between your breasts skin to your skin. Talk, sing, or provide your finger for sucking for comfort. Try to breastfeed again in a little while. Or, the baby may start moving to the breast on his or her own from this position.

Does your baby have a weak suck or make only tiny suckling movements? Break your baby's suction and try again. He or she may not have a deep enough latch to remove the milk from your breast. Talk with a lactation consultant or pediatrician if your baby's suck feels weak or if you are not sure he or she is getting enough milk. Rarely, a health problem causes the weak suck.

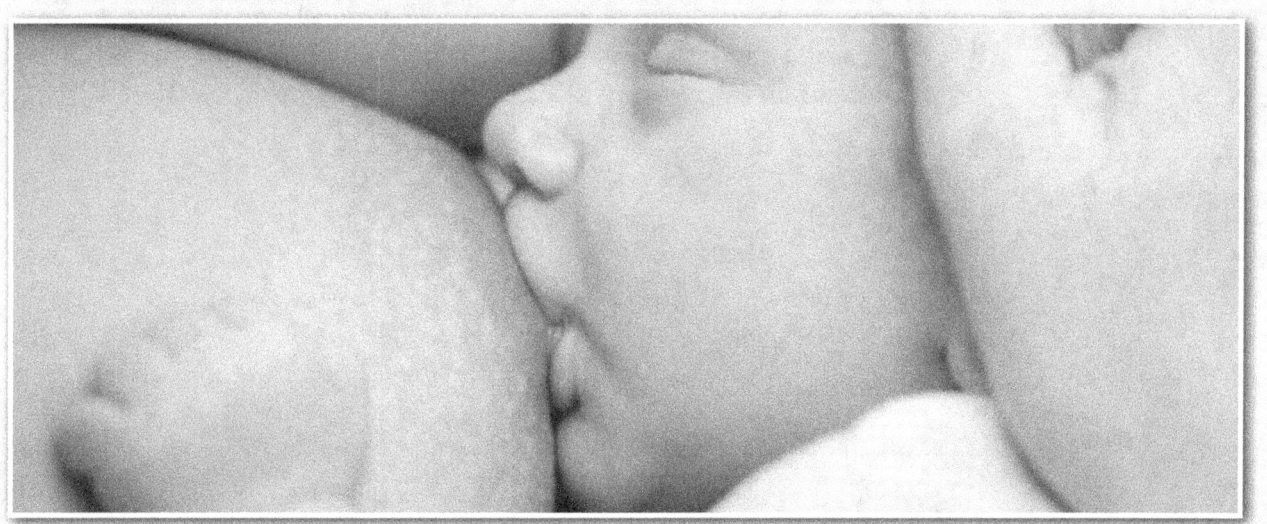

Breastfeeding Holds

Some moms find that the following positions are helpful ways to get comfortable and support their babies in finding a good latch. You also can use pillows under your arms, elbows, neck, or back to give you added comfort and support. Keep in mind that what works well for one feeding may not work well for the next. Keep trying different positions until you are comfortable.

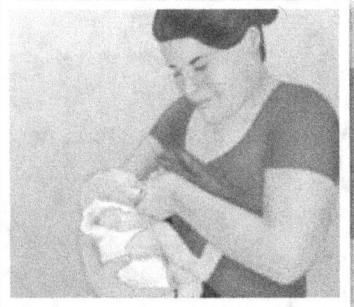

1. **Cradle hold** – an easy, common hold that is comfortable for most mothers and babies. Hold your baby with his or her head on your forearm and his or her whole body facing yours.

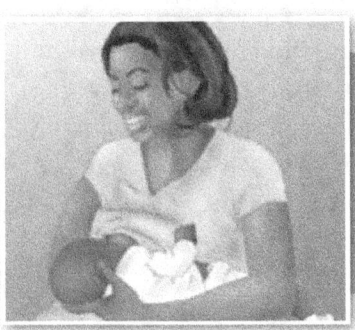

2. **Cross cradle or transitional hold** – useful for premature babies or babies with a weak suck because it gives extra head support and may help babies stay latched. Hold your baby along the opposite arm from the breast you are using. Support your baby's head with the palm of your hand at the base of his or her neck.

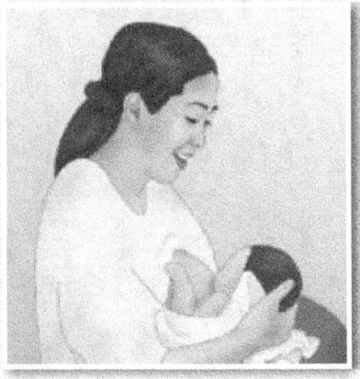

3. **Clutch or "football" hold** – useful for mothers who had a c-section and mothers with large breasts, flat or inverted nipples, or a strong let-down reflex (see **page 9**). It is also helpful for babies who prefer to be more upright. This hold allows you to better see and control your baby's head and to keep the baby away from a c-section incision. Hold your baby at your side, lying on his or her back, with his or her head at the level of your nipple. Support baby's head with the palm of your hand at the base of the head. (The baby is placed almost under the arm.)

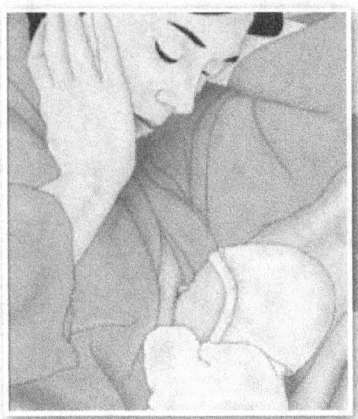

4. **Side-lying position** – useful for mothers who had a c-section or to help any mother get extra rest while the baby breastfeeds. Lie on your side with your baby facing you. Pull your baby close so your baby faces your body.

Tips for Making It Work

1. **Learn your baby's hunger signs.** When babies are hungry, they become more alert and active. They may put their hands or fists to their mouths, make sucking motions with their mouth, or turn their heads looking for the breast. If anything touches the baby's cheek – such as a hand – the baby may turn toward the hand, ready to eat. This sign of hunger is called rooting. Offer your breast when your baby shows rooting signs. Crying can be a late sign of hunger, and it may be harder to latch once the baby is upset. Over time, you will be able to learn your baby's cues for when to start feeding.

2. **Follow your baby's lead.** Make sure you are both comfortable and follow your baby's lead after he or she is latched on well. Some babies take both breasts at each feeding. Other babies only take one breast at a feeding. Help your baby finish the first breast, as long as he or she is still sucking and swallowing. This will ensure the baby gets the "hind" milk – the fattier milk at the end of a feeding. Your baby will let go of the breast when he or she is finished and often falls asleep. Offer the other breast if he or she seems to want more.

3. **Keep your baby close to you.** Remember that your baby is not used to this new world and needs to be held very close to his or her mother. Being skin to skin helps babies cry less and stabilizes the baby's heart and breathing rates.

How long should I breastfeed?

Many leading health organizations recommend that most infants breastfeed for at least 12 months, with exclusive breastfeeding for the first 6 months. This means that babies are not given any foods or liquids other than breast milk for the first 6 months. These recommendations are supported by organizations including the American Academy of Pediatrics, American Academy of Family Physicians, American College of Obstetricians and Gynecologists, American College of Nurse-Midwives, American Dietetic Association, and American Public Health Association.

Vitamin D

Babies need 400 IU of vitamin D each day. Ask your baby's doctor about supplements in drop form.

4. **Avoid nipple confusion.** Avoid using pacifiers, bottles, and supplements of infant formula in the first few weeks unless there is a medical reason to do so. If supplementation is needed, try to give expressed breast milk first. But it's best just to feed at the breast. This will help you make milk and keep your baby from getting confused while learning to breastfeed.

5. **Sleep safely and close by.** Have your baby sleep in a crib or bassinet in your room, so that you can breastfeed more easily at night. Sharing a room with parents is linked to a lower risk of SIDS (sudden infant death syndrome).

6. **Know when to wake the baby.** In the early weeks after birth, you should wake your baby to feed if 4 hours have passed since the beginning of the last feeding. Some tips for waking the baby include:

   - Changing your baby's diaper
   - Placing your baby skin to skin
   - Massaging your baby's back, abdomen, and legs

If your baby is falling asleep at the breast during most feedings, talk to the baby's doctor about a weight check. Also, see a lactation consultant to make sure the baby is latching on well.

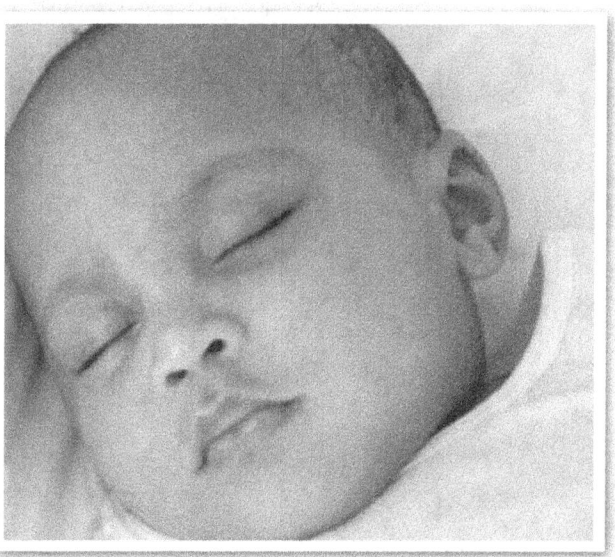

Making Plenty of Milk

Your breasts will easily make and supply milk directly in response to your baby's needs. The more often and effectively a baby breastfeeds, the more milk will be made. Babies are trying to double their weight in a few short months, and their tummies are small, so they need many feedings to grow and to be healthy.

Most mothers can make plenty of milk for their baby. If you think you have a low milk supply, talk to a lactation consultant. See **page 6** for other types of health professionals who can help you.

	What will happen with you, your baby, and your milk in the first few weeks		
Time	Milk	The Baby	You (Mom)
Birth	Your body makes colostrum (a rich, thick, yellowish milk) in small amounts. It gives your baby a healthy dose of early protection against diseases.	Will probably be awake in the first hour after birth. This is a good time to breastfeed your baby.	You will be tired and excited.
First 12-24 hours	Your baby will drink about 1 teaspoon of colostrum at each feeding. You may or may not see the colostrum, but it has what the baby needs and in the right amount.	It is normal for the baby to sleep heavily. Labor and delivery are hard work! Some babies like to nuzzle and may be too sleepy to latch well at first. Feedings may be short and disorganized. As your baby wakes up, take advantage of your baby's strong instinct to suck and feed every 1-2 hours. Many babies like to eat or lick, pause, savor, doze, then eat again.	You will be tired, too. Be sure to rest.
Next 3-5 days	Your white milk comes in. It is normal for it to have a yellow or golden tint first. Talk to a doctor and lactation consultant if your milk is not yet in.	Your baby will feed a lot (this helps your breasts make plenty of milk), at least 8-12 times or more in 24 hours. Very young breastfed babies don't eat on a schedule. Because breast milk is more easily digested than formula, breastfed babies eat more often than formula-fed babies. It is okay if your baby eats every 2-3 hours for several hours, then sleeps for 3-4 hours. Feedings may take about 15-20 minutes on each side. The baby's sucking rhythm will be slow and long. You might hear gulping.	Your breasts may feel full and leak. (You can use disposable or cloth pads in your bra to help with leaking.)
The first 4-6 weeks	White breast milk continues.	Your baby will likely be better at breastfeeding and have a larger stomach to hold more milk. Feedings may take less time and will be farther apart.	Your body gets used to breastfeeding so your breasts will be softer and the leaking may slow down.

How to Know Your Baby Is Getting Enough Milk

Many babies, but not all, lose a small amount of weight in the first days after birth. Your baby's doctor will check his or her weight at your first visit after you leave the hospital. Make sure to visit your baby's doctor within three to five days after birth and then again at two to three weeks of age for checkups.

You can tell if your baby is getting plenty of milk if he or she is mostly content and gaining weight steadily after the first week of age. From birth to three months, typical weight gain is 2/3 to 1 ounce each day.

Other signs that your baby is getting plenty of milk:

- He or she is passing enough clear or pale yellow urine, and it's not deep yellow or orange (see the chart below).
- He or she has enough bowel movements (see the chart below).
- He or she switches between short sleeping periods and wakeful, alert periods.
- He or she is satisfied and content after feedings.
- Your breasts feel softer after you feed your baby.

Talk to your baby's doctor if you are worried that your baby is not eating enough.

How much do babies typically eat?

A newborn's tummy is very small, especially in the early days. Once breastfeeding is established, exclusively breastfed babies from 1 to 6 months of age take in between 19 and 30 ounces per day. If you breastfeed 8 times per day, the baby would eat around 3 ounces per feeding. Older babies will take less breastmilk as other food is introduced. Every baby is different, though.

The Newborn Tummy

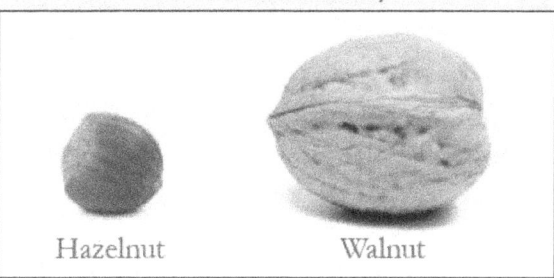

Hazelnut   Walnut

At birth, the baby's stomach can comfortably digest what would fit in a hazelnut (about 1-2 teaspoons). In the first week, the baby's stomach grows to hold about 2 ounces or what would fit in a walnut.

See our diaper tracker on page 46!

Minimum number of wet diapers and bowel movements in a baby's first week
(it is fine if your baby has more) 1 day = 24 hours

Baby's Age	Number of Wet Diapers	Number of Bowel Movements	Color and Texture of Bowel Movements
Day 1 (first 24 hours after birth)	1	The first one usually occurs within 8 hours after birth	Thick, tarry, and black
Day 2	2	3	Thick, tarry, and black
Day 3	5-6	3	Looser greenish to yellow (color may vary)
Day 4	6	3	Yellow, soft, and watery
Day 5	6	3	Loose and seedy, yellow color
Day 6	6	3	Loose and seedy, yellow color
Day 7	6	3	Larger amounts of loose and seedy, yellow color

Common Challenges

Breastfeeding can be challenging at times, especially in the early days. But it is important to remember that you are not alone. Lactation consultants are trained to help you find ways to make breastfeeding work for you. And while many women are faced with one or more of the challenges listed here, many women do not struggle at all! Also, many women may have certain problems with one baby that they don't have with their second or third babies. Read on for ways to troubleshoot problems.

Challenge: Sore Nipples

Many moms report that nipples can be tender at first. Breastfeeding should be comfortable once you have found some positions that work and a good latch is established. Yet it is possible to still have pain from an abrasion you already have. You may also have pain if your baby is sucking on only the nipple.

What you can do

1. A good latch is key, so see **page 13** for detailed instructions. If your baby is sucking only on the nipple, gently break your baby's suction to your breast by placing a clean finger in the corner of your baby's mouth and try again. (Your nipple should not look flat or compressed when it comes out of your baby's mouth. It should look round and long, or the same shape as it was before the feeding.)

2. If you find yourself wanting to delay feedings because of pain, get help from a lactation consultant. Delaying feedings can cause more pain and harm your supply.

3. Try changing positions each time you breastfeed. This puts the pressure on a different part of the breast.

4. After breastfeeding, express a few drops of milk and gently rub it on your nipples with clean hands. Human milk has natural healing properties and emollients that soothe. Also try letting your nipples air-dry after feeding, or wear a soft cotton shirt.

5. If you are thinking about using creams, hydrogel pads, or a nipple shield, get help from a health care provider first.

6. Avoid wearing bras or clothes that are too tight and put pressure on your nipples.

7. Change nursing pads often to avoid trapping in moisture.

8. Avoid using soap or ointments that contain astringents or other chemicals on your nipples. Make sure to avoid products that must be removed before breastfeeding. Washing with clean water is all that is needed to keep your nipples and breasts clean.

9. If you have very sore nipples, you can ask your doctor about using non-aspirin pain relievers.

Ask a lactation consultant for help to improve your baby's latch. Talk to your doctor if your pain does not go away or if you suddenly get sore nipples after several weeks of pain-free breastfeeding. Sore nipples may lead to a breast infection, which needs to be treated by a doctor.

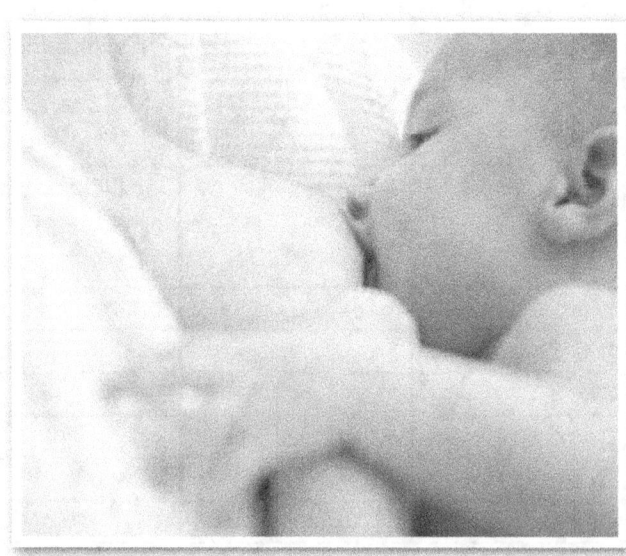

Challenge: Low Milk Supply

Most mothers can make plenty of milk for their babies. But many mothers are concerned about having enough.

Checking your baby's weight and growth is the best way to make sure he or she is getting enough milk. Let the doctor know if you are concerned. For more ways to tell if your baby is getting enough milk, see **page 17.**

There may be times when you think your supply is low, but it is actually just fine:

- When your baby is around six weeks to two months old, your breasts may no longer feel full. This is normal. At the same time, your baby may nurse for only five minutes at a time. This can mean that you and baby are just adjusting to the breastfeeding process – and getting good at it!

- Growth spurts can cause your baby to want to nurse longer and more often. These growth spurts can happen around two to three weeks, six weeks, and three months of age. They can also happen at any time. Don't be alarmed that your supply is too low to satisfy your baby. Follow your baby's lead – nursing more and more often will help build up your milk supply. Once your supply increases, you will likely be back to your usual routine.

What you can do

1. Make sure your baby is latched on and positioned well.

2. Breastfeed often and let your baby decide when to end the feeding.

3. Offer both breasts at each feeding. Have your baby stay at the first breast as long as he or she is still sucking and swallowing. Offer the second breast when the baby slows down or stops.

4. Try to avoid giving your baby formula or cereal as it may lead to less interest in breast milk. This will decrease your milk supply. Your baby doesn't need solid foods until he or she is at least six months old. If you need to supplement the baby's feedings, try using a spoon, cup, or a dropper.

5. Limit or stop pacifier use while trying the above tips at the same time.

Let your baby's doctor know if you think the baby is not getting enough milk.

Challenge: Oversupply of Milk

Some mothers are concerned about having an *oversupply* of milk. Having an overfull breast can make feedings stressful and uncomfortable for both mother and baby.

What you can do

1. Breastfeed on one side for each feeding. Continue to offer that same side for at least two hours until the next full feeding, gradually increasing the length of time per feeding.

2. If the other breast feels unbearably full before you are ready to breastfeed on it, hand express for a few moments to relieve some of the pressure. You can also use a cold compress or washcloth to reduce discomfort and swelling.

3. Feed your baby before he or she becomes overly hungry to prevent aggressive sucking. (Learn about hunger signs on **page 15.**)

4. Try positions that don't allow the force of gravity to help as much with milk ejection, such as the side-lying position or the football hold. (see **page 14** for illustrations of these positions.)

5. Burp your baby frequently if he or she is gassy.

Some women have a strong milk ejection reflex or let-down (see **page 9**). This can happen along with an oversupply of milk. If you have a rush of milk, try the following:

1. Hold your nipple between your forefinger and middle finger or with the side of your hand to

lightly compress milk ducts to reduce the force of the milk ejection.

2. If baby chokes or sputters, unlatch him or her and let the excess milk spray into a towel or cloth.

3. Allow your baby to come on and off the breast at will.

> Ask a lactation consultant for help if you are unable to manage an oversupply of milk on your own.

Challenge: Engorgement

It is normal for your breasts to become larger, heavier, and a little tender when they begin making more milk. Sometimes this fullness may turn into engorgement, when your breasts feel very hard and painful. You also may have breast swelling, tenderness, warmth, redness, throbbing, and flattening of the nipple. Engorgement sometimes also causes a low-grade fever and can be confused with a breast infection. Engorgement is the result of the milk building up. It usually happens during the third to fifth day after birth, but it can happen at any time.

Engorgement can lead to plugged ducts or a breast infection (see **page 21**), so it is important to try to prevent it before this happens. If treated properly, engorgement should resolve.

What you can do

1. Breastfeed often after birth, allowing the baby to feed as long as he or she likes, as long as he or she is latched on well and sucking effectively. In the early weeks after birth, you should wake your baby to feed if four hours have passed since the beginning of the last feeding.

2. Work with a lactation consultant to improve the baby's latch.

3. Breastfeed often on the affected side to remove the milk, keep it moving freely, and prevent the breast from becoming overly full.

4. Avoid overusing pacifiers and using bottles to supplement feedings.

5. Hand express or pump a little milk to first soften the breast, areola, and nipple before breastfeeding.

6. Massage the breast.

7. Use cold compresses in between feedings to help ease pain.

8. If you are returning to work, try to pump your milk on the same schedule that the baby breastfed at home. Or, you can pump at least every four hours.

9. Get enough rest, proper nutrition, and fluids.

10. Wear a well-fitting, supportive bra that is not too tight.

> Ask your lactation consultant or doctor for help if the engorgement lasts for two days or more.

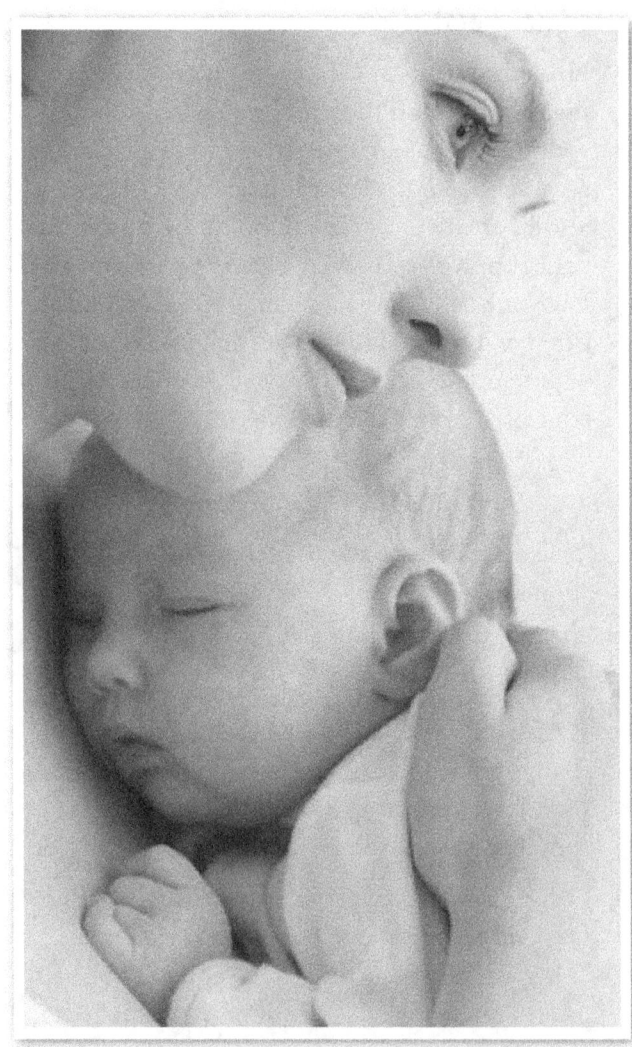

Challenge: Plugged Duct

It is common for many women to have a plugged duct at some point when breastfeeding. A plugged milk duct feels like a tender and sore lump in the breast. It is not accompanied by a fever or other symptoms. It happens when a milk duct does not properly drain and becomes inflamed. Then, pressure builds up behind the plug, and surrounding tissue becomes inflamed. A plugged duct usually only occurs in one breast at a time.

What you can do

1. Breastfeed often on the affected side, as often as every two hours. This helps loosen the plug, and keeps the milk moving freely.

2. Massage the area, starting behind the sore spot. Use your fingers in a circular motion and massage toward the nipple.

3. Use a warm compress on the sore area.

4. Get extra sleep or relax with your feet up to help speed healing. Often a plugged duct is the first sign that a mother is doing too much.

5. Wear a well-fitting supportive bra that is not too tight, because this can constrict milk ducts. Consider trying a bra without underwire.

If your plugged duct doesn't loosen up, ask for help from a lactation consultant. Plugged ducts can lead to a breast infection.

Challenge: Breast Infection (Mastitis)

Mastitis (mast-EYE-tiss) is soreness or a lump in the breast that can be accompanied by a fever and/or flu-like symptoms, such as feeling run down or very achy. Some women with a breast infection also have nausea and vomiting. You also may have yellowish discharge from the nipple that looks like colostrum. Or, the breasts may feel warm or hot to the touch and appear pink or red. A breast infection can occur when other family members have a cold or the flu. It usually only occurs in one breast. It is not always easy to tell the difference between a breast infection and a plugged duct because both have similar symptoms and can improve within 24 to 48 hours. Most breast infections that do not improve on their own within this time period need to be treated with medicine given by a doctor. (Learn more about medicines and breastfeeding on **page 26**.)

What you can do

1. Breastfeed often on the affected side, as often as every two hours. This keeps the milk moving freely and keeps the breast from becoming overly full.

2. Massage the area, starting behind the sore spot. Use your fingers in a circular motion and massage toward the nipple.

3. Apply heat to the sore area with a warm compress.

4. Get extra sleep or relax with your feet up to help speed healing. Often a breast infection is the first sign that a mother is doing too much and becoming overly tired.

5. Wear a well-fitting supportive bra that is not too tight, because this can constrict milk ducts.

Ask your doctor for help if you do not feel better within 24 hours of trying these tips, if you have a fever, or if your symptoms worsen. You might need medicine. **See your doctor right away if:**

- You have a breast infection in which both breasts look affected.
- There is pus or blood in the milk.
- You have red streaks near the area.
- Your symptoms came on severely and suddenly.

Even if you are taking medicine, continue to breastfeed during treatment. This is best for both you and your baby. Ask a lactation consultant for help if need be.

Challenge: Fungal Infections

A fungal infection, also called a yeast infection or thrush, can form on your nipples or in your breast because it thrives on milk. The infection forms from an overgrowth of the *Candida* organism. *Candida* exists in our bodies and is kept at healthy levels by the natural bacteria in our bodies. When the natural balance of bacteria is upset, *Candida* can overgrow, causing an infection.

A key sign of a fungal infection is if you develop sore nipples that last more than a few days, even after you make sure your baby has a good latch. Or, you may suddenly get sore nipples after several weeks of pain-free breastfeeding. Some other signs of a fungal infection include pink, flaky, shiny, itchy, or cracked nipples or deep pink and blistered nipples. You also could have achy breasts or shooting pains deep in the breast during or after feedings.

Causes of thrush include:

- Thrush in your baby's mouth, which can pass to you

- An overly moist environment on your skin or nipples that are sore or cracked

- Antibiotics or steroids

- A chronic illness like HIV, diabetes, or anemia

Thrush in a baby's mouth appears as little white spots on the inside of the cheeks, gums, or tongue. Many babies with thrush refuse to nurse or are gassy or cranky. A baby's fungal infection can also appear as a diaper rash that looks like small red dots around a main rash. This rash will not go away by using regular diaper rash creams.

What you can do

Fungal infections may take several weeks to cure, so it is important to follow these tips to avoid spreading the infection:

1. Change disposable nursing pads often.
2. Wash any towels or clothing that comes in contact with the yeast in very hot water (above 122°F).

3. Wear a clean bra every day.
4. Wash your hands often, and wash your baby's hands often – especially if he or she sucks on his or her fingers.
5. Put pacifiers, bottle nipples, or toys your baby puts in his or her mouth in a pot of water and bring it to a roaring boil daily. After one week of treatment, discard pacifiers and nipples and buy new ones.
6. Boil daily all breast pump parts that touch the milk.
7. Make sure other family members are free of thrush or other fungal infections. If they have symptoms, make sure they get treated.

If you or your baby has symptoms of a fungal infection, call both your doctor and your baby's doctor so you can be correctly diagnosed and treated at the same time. This will help prevent passing the infection to each other.

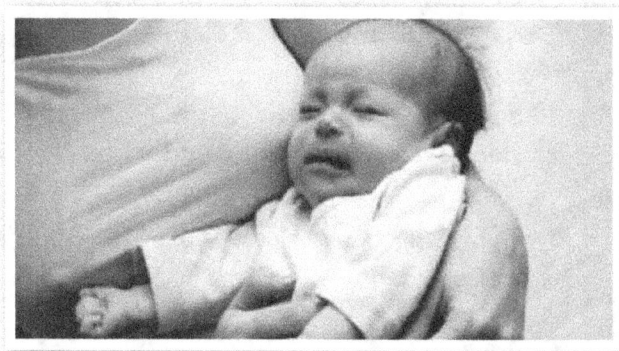

I had a terrible time learning to nurse my son. My nipples were terribly sore and it felt like it wasn't getting any better. After visiting my doctor, the lactation consultant, and the pediatrician, it became clear that a horrible case of thrush had been the source of my pain. I honestly did not think I would make it, but I was too stubborn to quit and I am grateful I stuck with it. I am proud to say that I breastfed my son until he was 16 months old!
– Jessica
Edmonton, AB, Canada

Challenge: Nursing Strike

A nursing "strike" is when your baby has been breastfeeding well for months and then suddenly begins to refuse the breast. A nursing strike can mean that your baby is trying to let you know that something is wrong. This does not usually mean that the baby is ready to wean. Not all babies will react the same to the different situations that can cause a nursing strike. Some babies will continue to breastfeed without a problem. Others may just become fussy at the breast, and others will refuse the breast entirely. Some of the major causes of a nursing strike include:

- Mouth pain from teething, a fungal infection like thrush, or a cold sore

- An ear infection, which causes pain while sucking

- Pain from a certain breastfeeding position, either from an injury on the baby's body or from soreness from an immunization

- Being upset about a long separation from the mother or a major change in routine

- Being distracted while breastfeeding – becoming interested in other things around him or her

- A cold or stuffy nose that makes breathing while breastfeeding difficult

- Reduced milk supply from supplementing with bottles or overuse of a pacifier

- Responding to the mother's strong reaction if the baby has bitten her

- Being upset after hearing people argue

- Reacting to stress, overstimulation, or having been repeatedly put off when wanting to breastfeed

If your baby is on a nursing strike, it is normal to feel frustrated and upset, especially if your baby is unhappy. It is important not to feel guilty or think that you have done something wrong. Keep in mind that your breasts may become uncomfortable as the milk builds up.

What you can do

1. Try to express your milk on the same schedule as the baby used to breastfeed to avoid engorgement and plugged ducts.

2. Try another feeding method temporarily to give your baby your milk, such as a cup, dropper, or spoon.

3. Keep track of your baby's wet diapers and dirty diapers to make sure he or she is getting enough milk.

4. Keep offering your breast to the baby. If the baby is frustrated, stop and try again later. You can also try when the baby is sleeping or very sleepy.

5. Try various breastfeeding positions, with your bare skin next to your baby's bare skin.

6. Focus on the baby with all of your attention and comfort him or her with extra touching and cuddling.

7. Try breastfeeding while rocking and in a quiet room free of distractions.

Ask for help if your baby is having a nursing strike to ensure that your baby gets enough milk. The doctor can check your baby's weight gain.

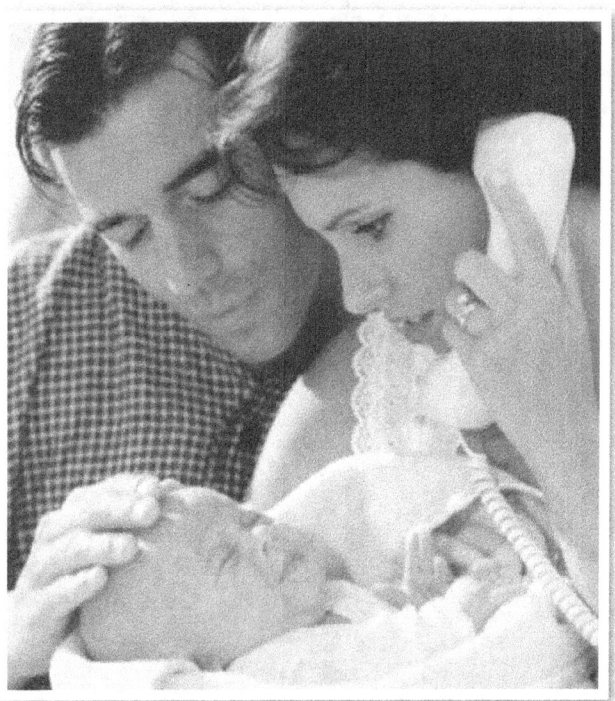

Challenge: Inverted, Flat, or Very Large Nipples

Some women have nipples that turn inward instead of protruding or that are flat and do not protrude. Nipples can also sometimes be flattened temporarily due to engorgement or swelling while breastfeeding. Inverted or flat nipples can sometimes make it harder to breastfeed. But remember that for breastfeeding to work, your baby has to latch on to both the nipple and the breast, so even inverted nipples can work just fine. Often, flat and inverted nipples will protrude more over time, as the baby sucks more.

Very large nipples can make it hard for the baby to get enough of the areola into his or her mouth to compress the milk ducts and get enough milk.

What you can do

1. Talk to your doctor or a lactation consultant if you are concerned about your nipples.

2. You can use your fingers to try and pull your nipples out. There are also special devices designed to pull out inverted or temporarily flattened nipples.

3. The latch for babies of mothers with very large nipples will improve with time as the baby grows. In some cases, it might take several weeks to get the baby to latch well. But if a mother has a good milk supply, her baby will get enough milk even with a poor latch.

Ask for help if you have questions about your nipple shape or type, especially if your baby is having trouble latching well.

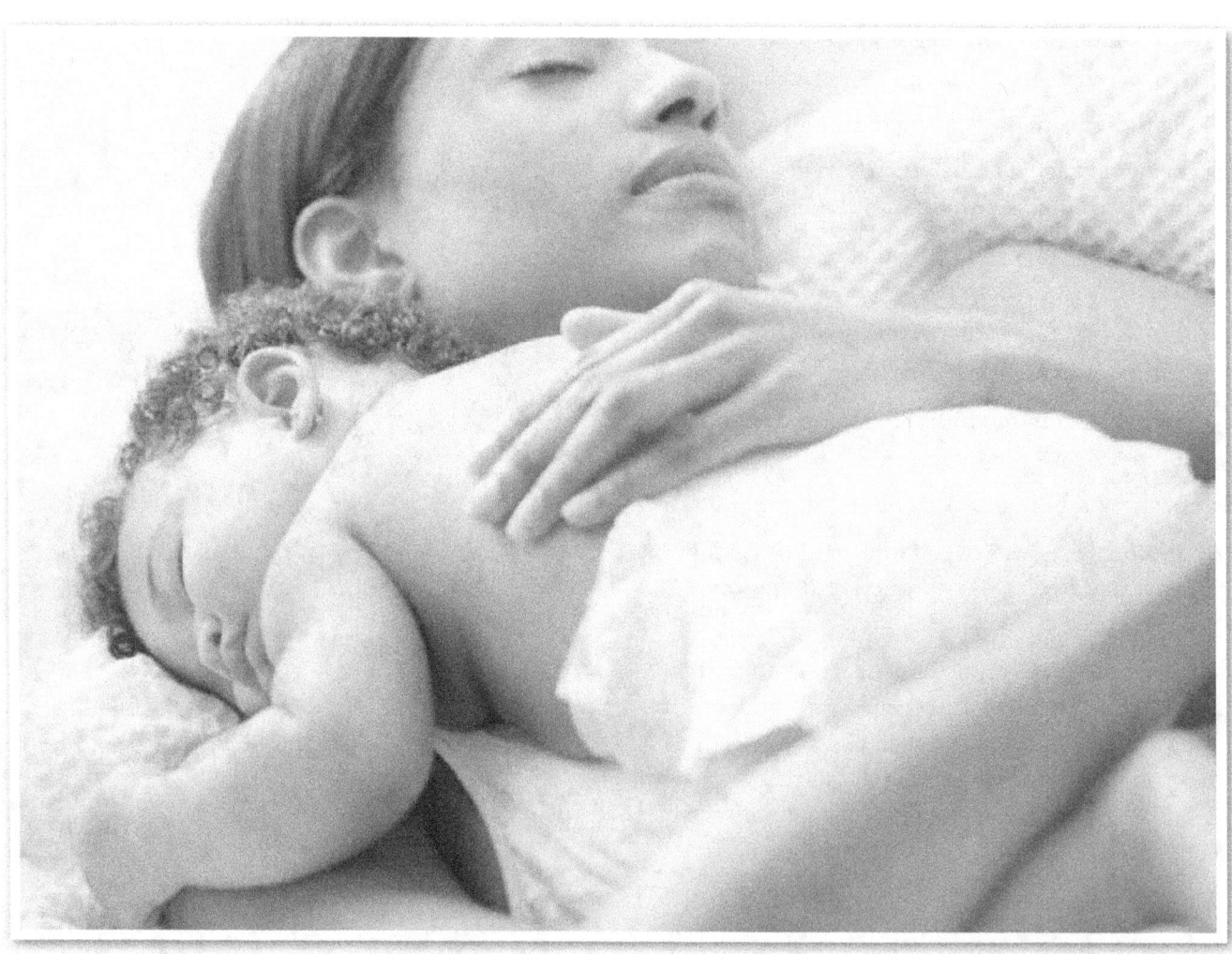

Common Questions

Should I supplement with formula?

Giving your baby formula may cause him or her to not want as much breast milk. This will decrease your milk supply. If you are worried that your baby is not eating enough, talk to your baby's doctor.

Does my baby need cereal or water?

Your baby only needs breast milk for the first six months of life. Breast milk alone will provide all the nutrition your baby needs. Giving the baby cereal may cause your baby to not want as much breast milk. This will decrease your milk supply. Even in hot climates, breastfed infants do not need water or juice. When your baby is ready for other foods, the food should be iron rich.

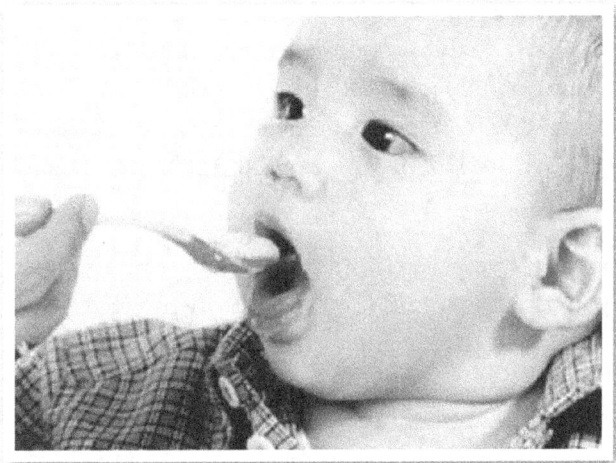

Is it okay for my baby to use a pacifier?

If you want to try it, it is best to wait until the baby is one month old to introduce a pacifier. This allows the baby to learn how to latch well on the breast and get enough to eat.

Is my baby getting enough vitamin D?

Vitamin D is needed to build strong bones. All infants and children should get at least 400 International Units (IU) of vitamin D each day. To meet this need, all breastfed infants (including those supplemented with formula) should be given a vitamin D supplement of 400 IU each day. This should start in the first few days of life. You can buy vitamin D supplements for infants at a drug store or grocery store. Sunlight is a major source of vitamin D, but it is hard to measure how much sunlight your baby gets, and too much sun can be harmful. Once your baby is weaned from breast milk, talk to your baby's doctor about whether your baby still needs vitamin D supplements. Some children do not get enough vitamin D through diet alone.

When should I wean my baby?

The American Academy of Pediatrics recommends breastfeeding beyond the baby's first birthday, and for as long as both the mother and baby would like. The easiest and most natural time to wean is when your child leads the process. But how the mother feels is very important in deciding when to wean.

Is it safe to smoke, drink, or use drugs?

If you smoke, it is best for you and your baby to quit as soon as possible. If you can't quit, it is still better to breastfeed because it can help protect your baby from respiratory problems and sudden infant death syndrome. Be sure to smoke away from your baby and change your clothes to keep your baby away from the chemicals smoking leaves behind. Ask a health care provider for help quitting smoking!

You should avoid alcohol, especially in large amounts. An occasional small drink is okay, but avoid breastfeeding for two hours after the drink.

It is not safe for you to use or be dependent on an illicit drug. Drugs such as cocaine, marijuana, heroine, and PCP harm your baby. Some reported side effects in babies include seizures, vomiting, poor feeding, and tremors.

Can I take medicines if I am breast-feeding?

Although almost all medicines pass into your milk in small amounts, most have no effect on the baby and can be used while breastfeeding. Very few medicines can't be used while breastfeeding. Discuss any medicines you are using with your doctor and ask before you start using new medicines. This includes prescription and over-the-counter drugs, vitamins, and dietary or herbal supplements. For some women with chronic health problems, stopping a medicine can be more dangerous than the effects it will have on the breastfed baby.

You can learn more from *Medications and Mothers' Milk,* a book by Thomas Hale, found in bookstores and libraries. The National Library of Medicine also offers an online tool for learning about the effects of medicines on breastfed babies. The website address is http://toxnet.nlm.nih.gov/cgi-bin/sis/htmlgen?LACT.

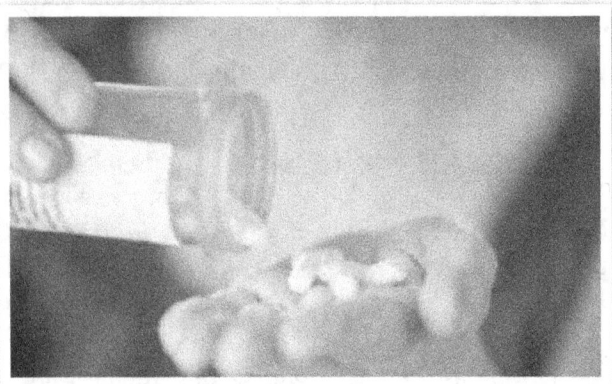

Can I breastfeed if I am sick?

Some women think that when they are sick, they should not breastfeed. But, most common illnesses, such as colds, flu, or diarrhea, can't be passed through breast milk. In fact, if you are sick, your breast milk will have antibodies in it. These antibodies will help protect your baby from getting the same sickness. (See **page 4** to learn about antibodies.)

Breastfeeding is not advised if the mother:

- Has been infected with HIV or has AIDS. If you have HIV and want to give your baby breast milk, you can contact a human milk bank (see page 32 for more information).

- Is taking antiretroviral medications.

- Has untreated, active tuberculosis.

- Is infected with human T-cell lymphotropic virus type I or type II.

- Is taking prescribed cancer chemotherapy agents, such as antimetabolites, that interfere with DNA replication and cell division.

- Is undergoing radiation therapies, but such nuclear medicine therapies require only a temporary break from breastfeeding.

What should I do if I have postpartum depression?

First, postpartum depression is different than postpartum "blues." The blues – which can include lots of tears, and feeling down and overwhelmed – are common and go away on their own. Postpartum depression is less common, more serious, and can last more than two weeks. Symptoms can include feeling irritable and sad, having no energy and not being able to sleep, being overly worried about the baby or not having interest in the baby, and feeling worthless and guilty.

If you have postpartum depression, work with your doctor to find the right treatment for you. Treatment may include medication such as antidepressants and talk therapy. Research has shown that while antidepressants pass into breast milk, few problems have been reported in infants. Even so, it is important to let your baby's doctor know if you need to take any medications.

Let your doctor know if your blues do not go away so that you can feel better. If you are having any thoughts about harming yourself or your baby, call 911 right away.

Will my partner be jealous if I breastfeed?

If you prepare your partner in advance, there should be no jealousy. Explain that you need support. Discuss the important and lasting health benefits of breastfeeding. Explain that not making formula means more rest. Be sure to emphasize that breastfeeding can save you money. Your partner can help by changing and burping the baby, sharing chores, and simply sitting with you and the baby to enjoy the special mood that breastfeeding creates. Your partner can also feed the baby pumped breast milk.

Do I have to restrict my sex life while breastfeeding?

No. But, if you are having vaginal dryness, you can try more foreplay and water-based lubricants. You can feed your baby or express some milk before lovemaking so your breasts will be more comfortable and less likely to leak. During sex, you also can put pressure on the nipple when it lets down or have a towel handy to catch the milk.

Do I still need birth control if I am breastfeeding?

Like other forms of birth control, breastfeeding is not a sure way to prevent pregnancy. Breastfeeding can delay the return of normal ovulation and menstrual cycles. You should still talk with a health care provider about birth control choices that are okay to use while breastfeeding.

I heard that breast milk can have toxins in it from my environment. Is it still safe for my baby?

While certain chemicals have appeared in breast milk, breastfeeding remains the best way to feed and nurture young infants and children. The advantages of breastfeeding far outweigh any possible risks from environmental pollutants. To date, the effects of such chemicals have only been seen rarely – in babies whose mothers themselves were ill because of them. Infant formula, the water it is mixed with, and/or the bottles or nipples used to give it to the baby can be contaminated with bacteria or chemicals.

Does my breastfed baby need vaccines? Is it safe for me to get a vaccine when I'm breastfeeding?

Yes. Vaccines are very important to your baby's health. Breastfeeding may also enhance your baby's response to certain immunizations, providing more protection. Follow the schedule your doctor gives you, and, if you miss any, check with him or her about getting your baby back on track. Breastfeeding while the vaccine is given to your baby – or immediately afterward – can help relieve pain and soothe an upset baby. Most nursing mothers may also receive vaccines. Breastfeeding does not affect the vaccine. Vaccines are not harmful to your breast milk.

What should I do if my baby bites me?

If your baby starts to clamp down, you can put your finger in the baby's mouth and take him or her off of your breast with a firm, "No." Try not to yell because it may scare the baby. If your baby continues to bite you, you can:

- Stop the feeding right away so the baby is not tempted to get another reaction from you. Don't laugh. This is part of your baby learning limits.

- Offer a teething toy, or a snack (if older baby), or drink from a cup instead.

- Put your baby down for a moment to show that biting brings a negative consequence. You can then pick your baby up again to give comfort.

What do I do if my baby keeps crying?

If your baby does not seem comforted by breastfeeding or other soothing measures, talk to your baby's doctor. Your baby may have colic or may be uncomfortable or in pain. You can also check to see if your baby is teething. The doctor and a lactation consultant can help you find ways to help your baby eat well.

Breastfeeding a Baby with Health Problems

There are some health problems in babies that can make it harder to breastfeed. Yet breast milk and early breastfeeding are still best for the health of both you and your baby – even more so if your baby is premature or sick. Even if your baby cannot breastfeed directly from you, it's best to express or pump your milk and give it to your baby with a cup or dropper.

Some common health problems in babies are listed below.

Jaundice

Jaundice (JAWN-diss) is caused by an excess of bilirubin, a substance that is in the blood usually in very small amounts. In the newborn period, bilirubin can build up faster than it can be removed from the intestinal track. Jaundice can appear as a yellowing of the skin and eyes. It affects most newborns to some degree, appearing between the second and third day of life. The jaundice usually clears up by two weeks of age and is not harmful.

Two types of jaundice can affect breastfed infants – breastfeeding jaundice and breast milk jaundice.

- Breastfeeding jaundice can occur when a breast-feeding baby is not getting enough breast milk. This can happen either because of breastfeeding challenges or because the mother's milk hasn't yet come in. This is not caused by a problem with the breast milk itself.

- Breast milk jaundice may be caused by substances in the mother's milk that prevents bilirubin from being excreted from the body. Such jaundice appears in some healthy, breastfed babies after about one week of age. It may last for a month or more and it is usually not harmful.

Your baby's doctor may monitor your baby's bilirubin level with blood tests. Jaundice is best treated by breastfeeding more frequently or for longer periods of time. It is crucial to have a health care provider help you make sure the baby is latching on and removing milk well. This is usually all that is needed for the infant's body to rid itself of excess bilirubin.

Some babies will also need phototherapy – treatment with a special light. This light helps break down bilirubin into a form that can be removed from the body easily. If you are having trouble latching your baby to the breast, it is important that you pump or hand express to ensure a good milk supply. The same is true if the baby needs formula for a short time – pumping or hand expressing will make sure the baby has enough milk when you return to breastfeeding.

It is important to keep in mind that breastfeeding is best for your baby. Even if your baby experiences jaundice, this is not something that you caused. Your health care providers can help you make sure that your baby is eating well and that the jaundice goes away.

> If your baby develops jaundice once at home, let your baby's doctor know. Discuss treatment options and let the doctor know that you do not want to interrupt breastfeeding if at all possible.

Reflux Disease

Some babies have a condition called gastroesophageal (GASS-troh-uh-SOF-uh-JEE-uhl) reflux disease (GERD), which occurs when the muscle at the opening of the stomach opens at the wrong times. This allows milk and food to come back up into the esophagus, the tube in the throat. Some symptoms of GERD can include:

- Severe spitting up, or spitting up after every feeding or hours after eating

- Projectile vomiting, where the milk shoots out of the mouth

- Inconsolable crying as if in discomfort

- Arching of the back as if in severe pain
- Refusal to eat or pulling away from the breast during feeding
- Waking up often at night
- Slow weight gain
- Gagging or choking, or problems swallowing

Many healthy babies might have some of these symptoms and not have GERD. But there are babies who might only have a few of these symptoms and have a severe case of GERD. Not all babies with GERD spit up or vomit. More severe cases of GERD may need to be treated with medication if the baby refuses to nurse, gains weight poorly or is losing weight, or has periods of gagging or choking.

See your baby's doctor if he or she spits up after every feeding and has any of the other symptoms mentioned here. If your baby has GERD, it is important to continue breastfeeding. Breast milk is more easily digested than infant formula.

Cleft Palate and Cleft Lip

Cleft palate and cleft lip are some of the most common birth defects that happen as a baby is developing in the womb. A cleft, or opening, in either the palate or lip can happen together or separately, and both can be corrected through surgery. Both conditions can prevent babies from forming a good seal around the nipple and areola with his or her mouth or effectively removing milk from the breast. A mother can try different breastfeeding positions and use her thumb or breast to help fill in the opening left by the lip to form a seal around the breast.

Right after birth, a mother whose baby has a cleft palate can try to breastfeed her baby. She can also start expressing her milk right away to keep up her supply. Even if her baby can't latch on well to her breast, the baby can be fed breast milk by cup. In some hospitals, babies with cleft palate are fitted with a mouthpiece called an obturator that fits into the cleft and seals it for easier feeding. The baby should be able to exclusively breastfeed after his or her surgery.

If your baby is born with a cleft palate or cleft lip, talk with a lactation consultant in the hospital. Breast milk is still best for your baby's health.

Premature and/or Low Birth Weight

Premature birth is when a baby is born before 37 weeks' gestation. Prematurity often will mean that the baby is born at a low birth weight, defined as less than 5½ pounds. Low birth weight can also be caused by malnourishment in the mother. Arriving early or being small can make for a tough adjustment, especially if the baby has to stay in the hospital for extra care. But keep in mind that breast milk has been shown to help premature babies grow and ward off illness.

Most babies who are low birth weight but born after 37 weeks (full term) can begin breastfeeding right away. They will need more skin-to-skin contact with mom and dad to help keep them warm. These smaller babies may also need more frequent feedings, and they may get sleepier during those feedings.

Many babies born prematurely are often not able to breastfeed at first, but they do benefit from expressed milk. You can express colostrum by hand or pump as soon as you can in the hospital. You can talk to the hospital staff about renting a hospital-grade electric pump. Call your insurance company or local WIC Office to find out if you can get reimbursed for this type of pump. You will need to express milk as often as you would have breastfed, so about 8 times in a 24-hour period.

Once your baby is ready to breastfeed directly, skin-to-skin contact can be very calming and a great start to your first feeding. Be sure to work with a lactation consultant on proper latch and positioning. Many mothers of premature babies find the cross cradle hold helpful. (See **page 14** for an illustration.) It may take some time for you and the baby to get into a good routine.

If you leave the hospital before your baby, you can express milk for the hospital staff to give the baby by feeding tube.

Breastfeeding and Special Situations

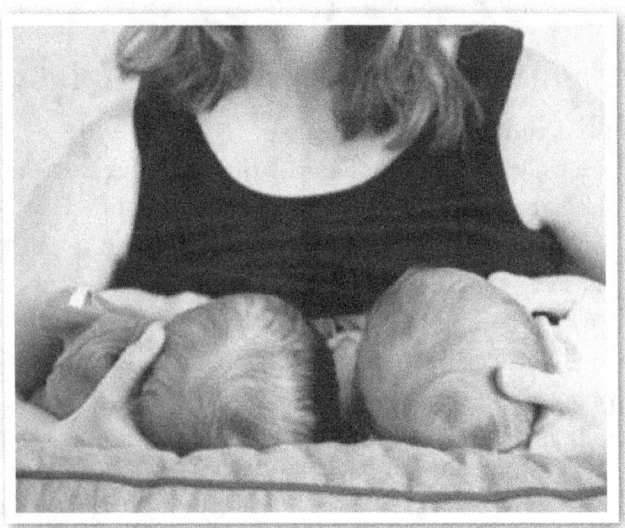

Twins or Multiples

The benefits of human milk to mothers of multiples and their babies are the same as for all mothers and babies – possibly greater, because many multiples are born early. But the idea may seem overwhelming! Yet many of these moms find breastfeeding easier than other feeding methods because there is nothing to prepare. Many mothers have overcome challenges to successfully breastfeed twins and more even after going back to work.

Being prepared

It will help to learn as much as you can about breastfeeding during your pregnancy. You can:

- Take a breastfeeding class.
- Find Internet and print resource for parents of multiples.
- Join a support group for parents of multiples

Many twin and multiple babies are smaller or born premature. Please see the information on **page 29** for other tips for caring for these babies. Also, talk with a lactation consultant about more ways you can successfully breastfeed.

through your health care provider, hospital, local breastfeeding center, or La Leche League International.

- Let your health care provider and family members know that you plan to breastfeed.
- Keep in mind that even if your babies need to spend time in the NICU (neonatal intensive care unit), breastfeeding is still possible, with some adjustments.
- Find a lactation consultant with multiples experience before the babies are born so that you know where to turn for help. Ask her where you can rent a breast pump if the babies are born early.

Making enough milk

Most mothers are able to make plenty of milk for twins. Many mothers fully breastfeed or provide milk for triplets or quadruplets. Keep these tips in mind:

- Breastfeeding soon after birth and often is helpful for multiples the same way it is for one baby. The more milk that is effectively removed, the more milk a mother's body will make.
- If the babies are born early, double pumping often will help the mother make more milk.
- The doctor's weight checks can tell you if your babies are getting enough breast milk. You can also track wet diapers and bowel movements to tell if your babies are getting enough. (See our diaper tracker on **page 46.**) For other signs that your babies are getting enough breast milk, see **page 17.**
- It helps to have each baby feed from both breasts. You can "assign" a breast to each baby for a feeding and switch at the next feeding. Or, you can assign a breast to each baby for a day and switch the next day. Switching breasts helps keep milk production up if one baby isn't eating as well for a bit. It also gives babies a different view to stimulate their eyes.

Breastfeeding positions

Breastfeeding twins and more may take practice, but you and your babies can find your ideal positions and routine. Keep trying different positions until you find ones that work for you. For some mothers and babies, breastfeeding twins at the same time works well. Others find individual feedings to work better. Still others find that it depends on the time – you may feed one baby at a time at night and feed two babies at the same time during the day. Finally, as your babies grow, you may find that you need to change your feeding routine.

Below are some positions that may work for you:

- **Double clutch** ("football") – Place both babies in the clutch hold. You will need pillows at your side (and maybe one on your lap) and you will place the babies on the pillows with their legs going toward the back of the chair or couch. If you are placing the babies in front of you, try to keep their whole bodies turned toward you, their chests against your chest. Their bodies must not be facing up. This is very important to help prevent nipple pain and to make sure that the babies are getting enough milk.

- **Cradle-clutch combination** – Place one baby (usually the easiest to latch or stay latched) in the cradle position and then position the second baby in the clutch position.

- **Double cradle** – Place the babies in front of you with their legs overlapping, making an X across your lap.

Partial breastfeeding

Even though full, direct breastfeeding is ideal, many mothers of multiples feed their babies breast milk or some formula by bottles at times. It is important to work with your doctor, your baby's doctor, and a lactation consultant to figure out what works best for your family.

Many breastfeeding basics are the same for twins or multiples as they are for one baby. Learn more about these important topics:

- How to know your babies are getting enough milk **(page 17)**

- How to troubleshoot common challenges **(page 18)**

- Ways to keep milk supply up **(page 19)**

Breastfeeding During Pregnancy

Breastfeeding during your next pregnancy is not a risk to either the breastfeeding toddler or to the new developing baby. If you are having some problems in your pregnancy such as uterine pain or bleeding, a history of preterm labor, or problems gaining weight during pregnancy, your doctor may advise you to wean. Some women also choose to wean at this time because they have nipple soreness caused by pregnancy hormones, are nauseous, or find that their growing bellies make breastfeeding uncomfortable. Your toddler also may decide to wean on his or her own because of changes in the amount and flavor of your milk. He or she will need additional food and drink because you will likely make less milk during pregnancy.

If you keep nursing your toddler after your baby is born, you can feed your newborn first to ensure he or she gets the colostrum. Once your milk production increases a few days after birth, you can decide how to best meet everyone's needs, especially the new baby's needs for you and your milk. You may want to ask your partner to help you by taking care of one child while you are breastfeeding. Also, you will have a need for more fluids, healthy foods, and rest because you are taking care of yourself and two small children.

Breastfeeding After Breast Surgery

How much milk you can produce depends on how your surgery was done and where your incisions are, and the reasons for your surgery. Women who have had incisions in the fold under the breasts are less likely to have problems making milk than women who have had incisions around or across the areola, which can cut into milk ducts and nerves. Women who have had breast implants usually breastfeed successfully. If you ever had surgery on your breasts for any reason, talk with a lactation consultant. If you are planning breast surgery, talk with your surgeon about ways he or she can preserve as much of the breast tissue and milk ducts as possible.

Adoption and Inducing Lactation

Many mothers who adopt want to breastfeed their babies and can do it successfully with some help. Many will need to supplement their breast milk with donated breast milk from a milk bank or infant formula, but some adoptive mothers can breastfeed exclusively, especially if they have been pregnant before. Lactation is a hormonal response to a physical action, and so the stimulation of the baby nursing causes the body to see a need for and produce milk. The more the baby nurses, the more a woman's body will produce milk.

If you are adopting and want to breastfeed, talk with both your doctor and a lactation consultant. They can help you decide the best way to try to establish a milk supply for your new baby. You might be able to prepare by pumping every three hours around the clock for two to three weeks before your baby arrives, or you can wait until the baby arrives and start to breastfeed then. Devices such as a supplemental nursing system (SNS) or a lactation aid can help ensure that your baby gets enough nutrition and that your breasts are stimulated to produce milk at the same time.

Using Milk from Donor Banks

If you can't breastfeed and still want to give your baby human milk, the best and only safe place to go is to a human milk bank. You should never feed your baby breast milk that you get directly from another woman or through the Internet. A human milk bank can dispense donor human milk to you if you have a prescription from your doctor. Many steps are taken to ensure the milk is safe. Donor human milk provides the same precious nutrition and disease-fighting properties as your own breast milk.

If your baby was born premature or has other health problems, he or she may need donated milk not only for health but also for survival. Your baby may also need donated milk if she or he:

- Can't tolerate formula
- Has severe allergies
- Isn't thriving on formula

You can find a human milk bank through the Human Milk Banking Association of North America (HMBANA). HMBANA is a multidisciplinary group of health care providers that promotes, protects, and supports donor milk banking. HMBANA is the only professional membership association for milk banks in Canada, Mexico, and the United States and as such sets the standards and guidelines for donor milk banking for those areas. You can also contact HMBANA if you would like to donate breast milk.

To find out if your insurance will cover the cost of the milk, call your insurance company or ask your doctor. If your insurance company does not cover the cost of the milk, talk with the milk bank to find out how payment can be made later on, or how to get help with the payments. A milk bank will never deny donor milk to a baby in need if it has the supply.

Breastfeeding in Public

Many women have reported feeling uncomfortable breastfeeding in public, even doing so discreetly. But it is important to remember that you are feeding your baby. You are not doing anything inappropriate. And even though it may seem taboo in some places, awareness of the need to support new breastfeeding mothers is building.

The federal government and many states have laws that protect nursing women. These laws are based on the recognition of organizations such as the American Academy of Pediatrics, the American College of Obstetricians and Gynecologists, American Public Health Association, United Nations International Children's Emergency Fund (UNICEF), and the World Health Organization (WHO) that breastfeeding is the best choice for the health of a mother and her baby.

Even with the growing awareness of the benefits of breastfeeding, you may find it difficult to do so in public. Yet it is important to believe in yourself and your choice. Remind yourself that you can succeed and wear your confidence! Some tips for breastfeeding in public include:

- Wear clothes that allow easy access to your breasts, such as tops that pull up from the waist or button down.

- Use a special breastfeeding blanket around your shoulders. Some babies do not like this, though, so you'll have to see what works for your baby.

- Breastfeed your baby in a sling. Slings or other soft infant carriers are especially helpful for traveling – it makes it easier to keep your baby comforted and close to you.

- Slip into a women's lounge or dressing room to breastfeed.

Follow the instructions for infant slings very carefully. Check in with the Consumer Product Safety Commission for warnings before buying a sling.

- If you are worried about being too revealing in public, practice at home until you are comfortable.

It helps to breastfeed your baby before he or she becomes fussy so that you have time to get into a comfortable place or position to feed. (Over time, you will learn your baby's early hunger cues.) When you get to your destination, scout out a place you can breastfeed, if that makes you feel more comfortable.

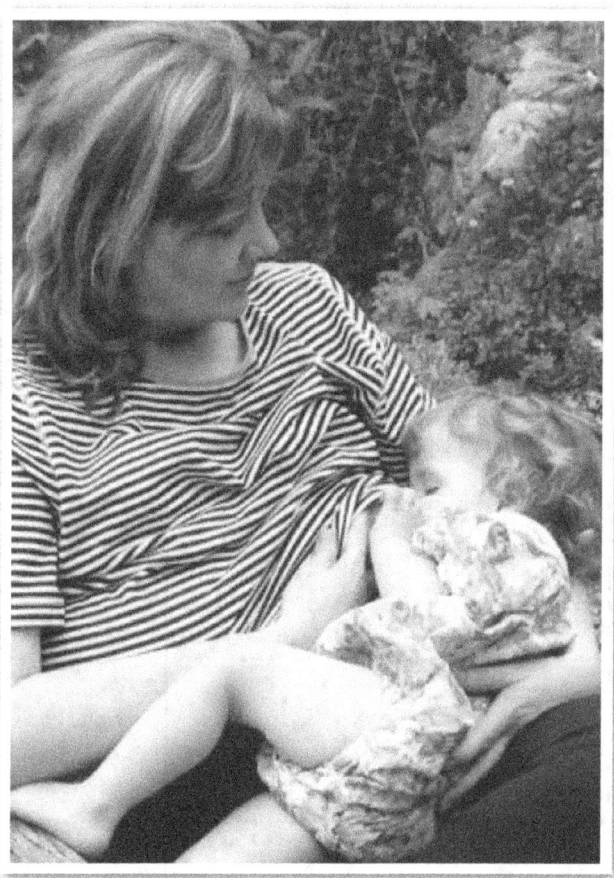

If someone criticizes you for breastfeeding in public, check out the La Leche League's website at http://www.llli.org for possible ways to respond.

Most of all, it is important to remember that you are meeting your baby's needs. It isn't possible to stay home all the time, and you can feel free to feed your baby while out and about. You should be proud of your commitment! Plus, no bottles and formula means fewer supplies to pack!

Pumping and Milk Storage

If you are unable to breastfeed your baby directly, it is important to remove milk during the times your baby normally would feed. This will help you continue to make milk. Before you express breast milk, be sure to wash your hands. Also, make sure the area where you are expressing is clean.

If you need help to get your milk to start flowing, have one of the following items nearby – a picture of your baby, a baby blanket, or an item of your baby's clothing that has his or her scent on it. You can also apply a warm moist compress to the breast, gently massage the breasts, or sit quietly and think of a relaxing setting.

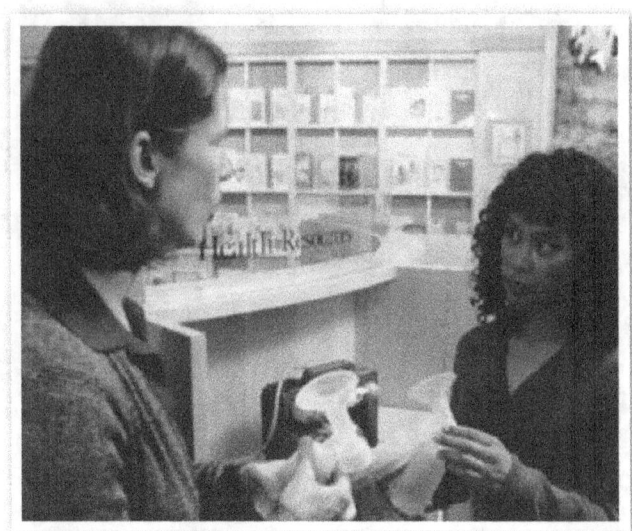

Ways to Express Your Milk			
Type	How It Works	What's Involved	Average Cost
Hand Expression	You use your hand to massage and compress your breast to remove milk.	• Requires practice, skill, and coordination. • Gets easier with practice; can be as fast as pumping. • Good if you are seldom away from baby or need an option that is always with you. But all moms should learn how to hand express.	Free, unless you need help from a breastfeeding professional who charges for her services.
Manual Pump	You use your hand and wrist to operate a hand-held device to pump the milk.	• Requires practice, skill, and coordination. • Useful for occasional pumping if you are away from baby once in a while.	$30 to $50
Automatic, Electric Breast Pump	Runs on battery or plugs into an electrical outlet.	• Can be easier for some moms. • Can pump one breast at a time or both breasts at the same time. • Double pumping may collect more milk in less time, so it is helpful if you are going back to work or school full time. • Need places to clean and store the equipment between uses.	$150 to over $250

Hospital-grade electric pumps can be rented from a lactation consultant at a local hospital or from a breastfeeding organization. These pumps work well for establishing milk supply when new babies can't feed at the breast. Mothers who have struggled with other expression methods may find that these pumps work well for them.

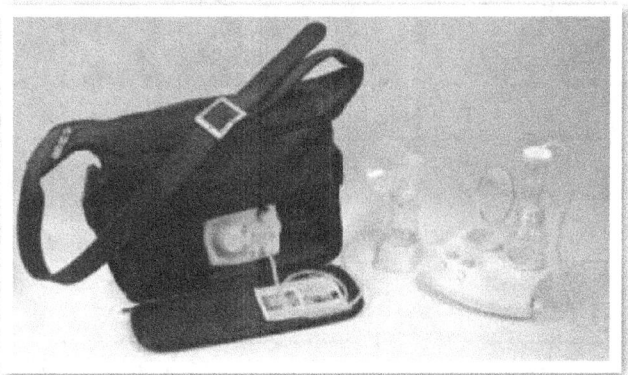

Electric Pumps

You can keep germs from getting into the milk by washing your pumping equipment with soap and water and letting it air dry.

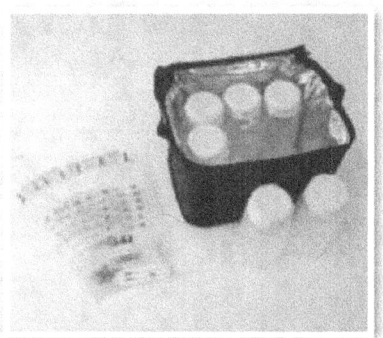
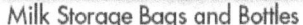

Milk Storage Bags and Bottles

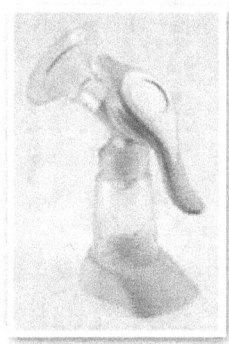

Manual Pump

Storage of Breast Milk

Breast milk can be stored in clean glass or hard BPA-free plastic bottles with tight-fitting lids. You can also use milk storage bags, which are made for freezing human milk. Do not use disposable bottle liners or other plastic bags to store breast milk.

After each pumping

- Label the date on the storage container. Include your child's name if you are giving the milk to a childcare provider.

- Gently swirl the container to mix the cream part of the breast milk that may rise to the top back into the rest of the milk. Shaking the milk is not recommended – this can cause a breakdown of some of the milk's valuable components.

- Refrigerate or chill milk right after it is expressed. You can put it in the refrigerator, place it in a cooler or insulated cooler pack, or freeze it in small (2 to 4 ounce) batches for later feedings.

Tips for freezing milk

- Wait to tighten bottle caps or lids until the milk is completely frozen.

- Try to leave an inch or so from the milk to the top of the container because it will expand when freezing.

- Store milk in the back of the freezer – not in the freezer door.

Tips for thawing and warming up milk

- Clearly label milk containers with the date it was expressed. Use the oldest stored milk first.

- Breast milk does not necessarily need to be warmed. Some moms prefer to take the chill off and serve at room temperature. Some moms serve it cold.

- Thaw frozen milk in the refrigerator overnight, by holding the bottle or frozen bag of milk under warm running water, or setting it in a container of warm water.

- Never put a bottle or bag of breast milk in the microwave. Microwaving creates hot spots that could burn your baby and damage the components of the milk.

- Swirl the milk and test the temperature by dropping some on your wrist. It should be comfortably warm.

- Use thawed breast milk within 24 hours. Do not re-freeze thawed breast milk.

Guide to Storing Fresh Breast Milk for Use with Healthy Full-Term Infants

Place	Temperature	How Long	Things to Know
Countertop, table	Room temp (60°F-85°F)	Up to 3-4 hours is best. Up to 6-8 hours is okay for very clean expressed milk.	Containers should be covered and kept as cool as possible; covering the container with a clean cool towel may keep milk cooler. Throw out any leftover milk within 1 to 2 hours after the baby is finished feeding.
Small cooler with a blue-ice pack.	59°F	24 hours.	Keep ice packs in contact with milk containers at all times; limit opening cooler bag.
Refrigerator	39°F or colder	Up to 72 hours is best. Up to 5-8 days is okay for very clean expressed milk.	Store milk in the back of the main body of the refrigerator.
Freezer	24°F or colder	Up to 6 months is best. Up to 12 months is okay if milk is stored at 0°F or colder.	Store milk toward the back of the freezer where temperature is most constant. Milk stored at 0°F or colder is safe for longer durations, but the quality of the milk might not be as high.

Guide to Storing Thawed Breast Milk

	Room Temperature (60°F to 85°F)	Refrigerator (39°F or colder)	Any Freezers
Thawed Breast Milk	Up to 1-2 hours is best. Up to 3-4 hours is okay.	24 hours	Do not re-freeze.

I was committed to breastfeeding, but learning to nurse while learning to take care of a newborn was tough. My baby hated taking the entire nipple, and slipping off as she nursed was painful. And when it's 3 a.m. and your baby is fussing and you are sore, those bottles are incredibly tempting.

At the same time, most of the health professionals I came in contact with – as well as many of my family members and friends – seemed to be undermining my breastfeeding relationship. My daycare providers seemed afraid of my breast milk, my workplace didn't offer me a place to pump, and other mothers would act as though my breastfeeding was condemning their choice not to.

But I remembered that my nurse, Charlene, asked me to give it at least 8 weeks. I remembered that advice and decided to wait a little longer. I went back to Charlene for help and she showed me how to combat my daughter's slipping latch. She also put me in touch with a local support group and helped me find professionals who really knew how to help. They got me through the most critical period, but it was only my willingness to seek out their guidance that allowed me to keep nursing. Don't be afraid to ask for help whenever you need it!

– Lin
Lock Haven, PA

Going Back to Work

Planning ahead for your return to work can help ease the transition. Learn as much as you can ahead of time and talk with your employer about your options. This can help you continue to enjoy breastfeeding your baby long after your maternity leave is over.

During Pregnancy

- Join a breastfeeding support group to talk with other mothers about breastfeeding while working.

- Talk with your supervisor about your plans to breastfeed. Discuss different types of schedules, such as starting back part time at first or taking split shifts.

- Find out if your company provides a lactation support program for employees. If not, ask about private areas where you can comfortably and safely express milk. The Affordable Care Act (health care reform) supports work-based efforts to assist nursing mothers.

- Ask the lactation program director, your supervisor, wellness program director, employee human resources office, or other coworkers if they know of other women at your company who have breastfed after returning to work.

After the Baby Is Born

- Follow the steps on **page 15** to set up a breastfeeding routine that works for you and your baby.

- Ask for help from a lactation consultant or your doctor, if you need it.

During Your Maternity Leave

- Take as many weeks off as you can. At least six weeks of leave can help you recover from childbirth and settle into a good breastfeeding routine. Twelve weeks is even better.

- Practice expressing your milk by hand or with a quality breast pump. Freeze 2 to 4 ounces at a time to save for your baby after you return to work. See **pages 34-36** for more information about pumping and storage.

- Help your baby adjust to taking breast milk from a bottle (or cup for infants 3 to 4 months old) shortly before you return to work. Babies are used to nursing with mom, so they usually drink from a bottle or cup when it's given by somebody else.

- See if there is a childcare option close to work, so that you can visit and breastfeed your baby, if possible. Ask if the facility will use your pumped breast milk.

- Talk with your family and your childcare provider about your desire to breastfeed. Let them know that you will need their support.

Back at Work

- Keep talking with your supervisor about your schedule and what is or isn't working for you. Keep in mind that returning to work gradually gives you more time to adjust.

- If your childcare is close by, find out if you can visit to breastfeed over lunch.

- When you arrive to pick up your baby from childcare, take time to breastfeed first. This will give you both time to reconnect before traveling home and returning to other family responsibilities.

- If you are having a hard time getting support, talk to your human resources department. You can also ask a lactation consultant for tips.

Get a Quality Breast Pump

A good-quality electric breast pump may be your best strategy for efficiently removing milk during the workday. Contact a lactation consultant or your local hospital, WIC program, or public health department to learn where to buy or rent a good pump. Electric pumps that allow you to express milk from both breasts at the same time reduce pumping time.

Find a Private Place to Express Milk

Work with your supervisor to find a private place to express your milk. The Affordable Care Act (health care reform) supports work-based efforts to assist nursing mothers. The Department of Labor is proposing a new regulation to allow nursing women reasonable break time in a private place (other than a bathroom) to express milk while at work. (Employers with fewer than 50 employees are not required to comply if it would cause the company financial strain.)

If your company does not provide a private lactation room, find another private area you can use. You may be able to use:

- An office with a door
- A conference room
- A little-used closet or storage area

The room should be private and secure from intruders when in use. The room should also have an electrical outlet if you are using an electric breast pump. Explain to your supervisor that it is best not to express milk in a restroom. Restrooms are unsanitary, and there are usually no electrical outlets. It can also be difficult to manage a pump in a toilet stall.

Pumping Tips

It may take time to adjust to pumping breast milk in a work environment. For easier pumping, try these tips for getting your milk to let-down from the milk ducts:

- Relax as much as you can
- Massage your breasts
- Gently rub your nipples
- Visualize the milk flowing down
- Think about your baby – bring a photo of your baby, or a blanket or item of clothing that smells like your baby

When to Express Milk

At work, you will need to express and store milk during the times you would normally feed your baby. (In the first few months of life, babies need to breastfeed 8 to 12 times in 24 hours.) This turns out to be about 2 to 3 times during a typical 8-hour work period. Expressing milk can take about 10 to 15 minutes. Sometimes it may take longer. This will help you make enough milk for your childcare provider to feed your baby while you are at work. The number of times you need to express milk at work should be equal to the number of feedings your baby will need while you are away. As the baby gets older, the number of feeding times may go down. Many women take their regular breaks and lunch breaks to pump. Some women come to work early or stay late to make up the time needed to express milk.

Storing Your Milk

Breast milk is food, so it is safe to keep it in an employee refrigerator or a cooler with ice packs. Talk to your supervisor about the best place to store your milk. If you work in a medical department, do not store milk in the same refrigerators where medical specimens are kept. Be sure to label the milk container with your name and the date you expressed the milk.

Call to Action to Support Breastfeeding

The Surgeon General's Call to Action to Support Breastfeeding explains why breastfeeding is a national public health priority and sets forth actionable steps that businesses, communities, health systems, and others can take to support nursing mothers. Learn more at http://www.surgeongeneral.gov.

The Business Case for Breastfeeding is a resource kit that can help your company support you and other breastfeeding mothers in the workplace. Share this website with your supervisor: http://www.womenshealth.gov/breastfeeding/government-programs/business-case-for-breastfeeding.

Nutrition and Fitness

Healthy Eating

Many new mothers wonder if they should be on a special diet while breastfeeding, but the answer is no. You can take in the same number of calories that you did before becoming pregnant, which helps with weight loss after birth. There are no foods you have to avoid. In fact, you can continue to enjoy the foods that are important to your family – the special meals you know and love.

As for how your diet affects your baby, there are no special foods that will help you make more milk. You may find that some foods cause stomach upset in your baby. You can try avoiding those foods to see if your baby feels better and ask your baby's doctor for help.

Keep these important nutrition tips in mind:

• Drink plenty of fluids to stay hydrated (but fluid intake does not affect the amount of breast milk you make). Drink when you are thirsty, and drink more fluids if your urine is dark yellow. A common suggestion is to drink a glass of water or other beverage every time you breastfeed. Limit beverages that contain added sugars, such as soft drinks and fruit drinks.

• Drinking a moderate amount (up to 2 to 3 cups a day) of coffee or other caffeinated beverages does not cause a problem for most breastfeeding babies. Too much caffeine can cause the baby to be fussy or not sleep well.

• Vitamin and mineral supplements cannot replace a healthy diet. In addition to healthy food choices, some breastfeeding women may need a multivitamin and mineral supplement. Talk with your doctor to find out if you need a supplement.

• See **page 25** for information on drinking alcohol and breastfeeding.

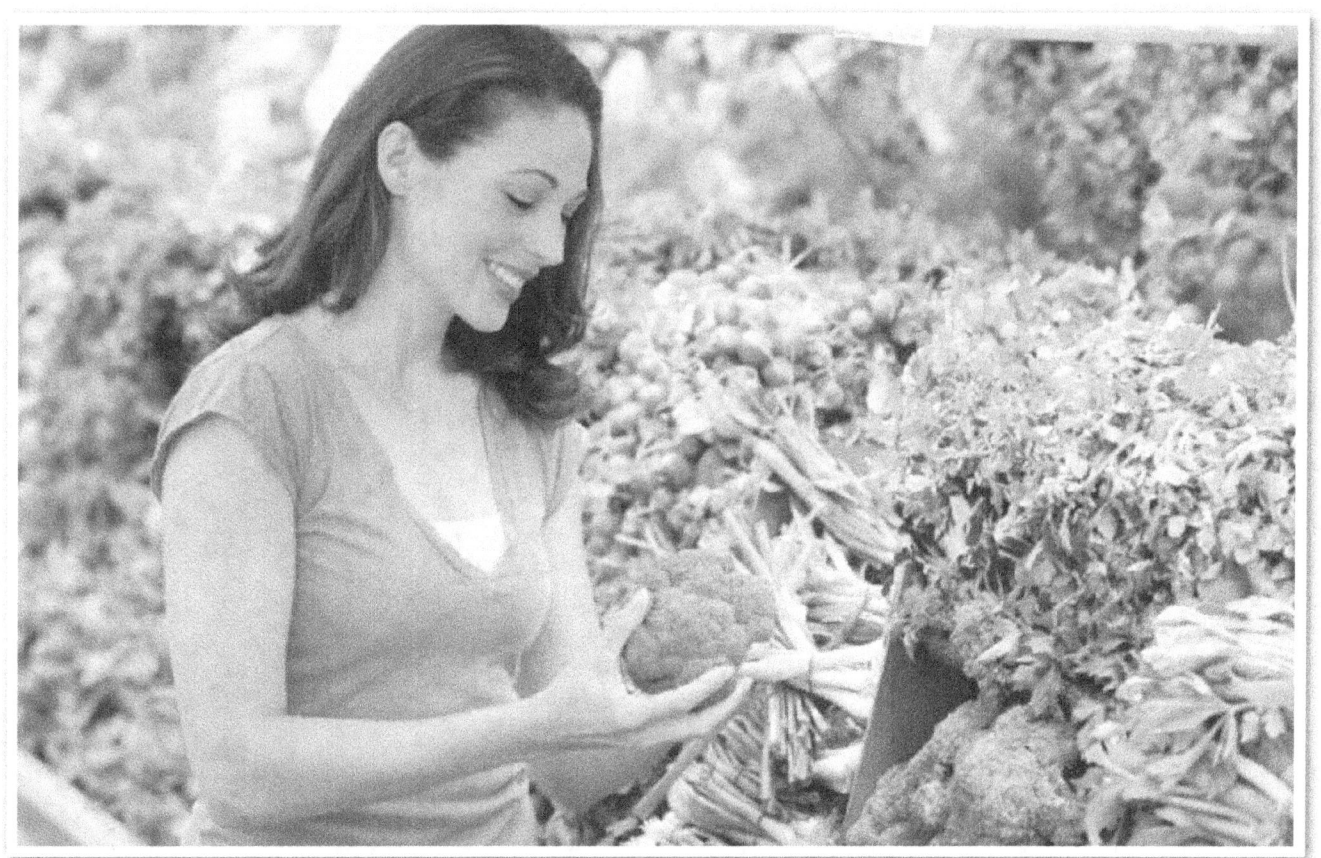

Can a baby be allergic to breast milk?

Research shows that a mother's milk is affected only slightly by the foods she eats. Breastfeeding mothers can eat whatever they have eaten during their lifetimes and do not need to avoid certain foods. Babies love the flavors of foods that come through in your milk. Sometimes a baby may be sensitive to something you eat, such as dairy products like milk and cheese. Symptoms in your baby of an allergy or sensitivity to something you eat include some or all of these:

- Green stools with mucus and/or blood, diarrhea, vomiting
- Rash, eczema (EG-zuh-muh), dermatitis, hives, dry skin
- Fussiness during and/or after feedings
- Crying for long periods without being able to feel consoled
- Sudden waking with discomfort
- Wheezing or coughing

Babies who are highly sensitive usually react to the food the mother eats within minutes or within 4 to 24 hours afterward. These signs do not mean the baby is allergic to your milk itself, only to something you are eating. If you stop eating whatever is bothering your baby or eat less of it, the problem usually goes away on its own. You also can talk with your baby's doctor about any symptoms. If your baby ever has problems breathing, call 911 or go to your nearest emergency room.

MyPyramid Plans for Moms

The USDA's online, interactive tool can help you choose foods based on your baby's nursing habits and your energy needs. Visit http://www.mypyramid.gov/mypyramidmoms/pyramidmoms_plan.aspx to:

- Figure out how much you need to eat
- Choose healthy foods
- Get the vitamins and minerals you need

For a sample of nutrition needs for breastfeeding mothers, see **page 41**.

Vegan diets

If you follow a vegan diet or one that does not include any forms of animal protein, you or your baby might not get enough vitamin B12 in your bodies. This can also happen if you eat meat, but not enough. In a baby, this can cause symptoms such as loss of appetite, slow motor development, being very tired, weak muscles, vomiting, and blood problems. You can protect your and your baby's health by taking vitamin B12 supplements while breastfeeding. Talk to your doctor about your vitamin B12 needs.

Fitness

An active lifestyle helps you stay healthy, feel better, and have more energy. It does not affect the quality or quantity of your breast milk or your baby's growth. If your breasts are large or heavy, it may help to wear a comfortable support bra or sports bra and pads in case you leak during exercise. It is also important to drink plenty of fluids. Be sure to talk to your doctor about how and when to slowly begin exercising after your baby's birth.

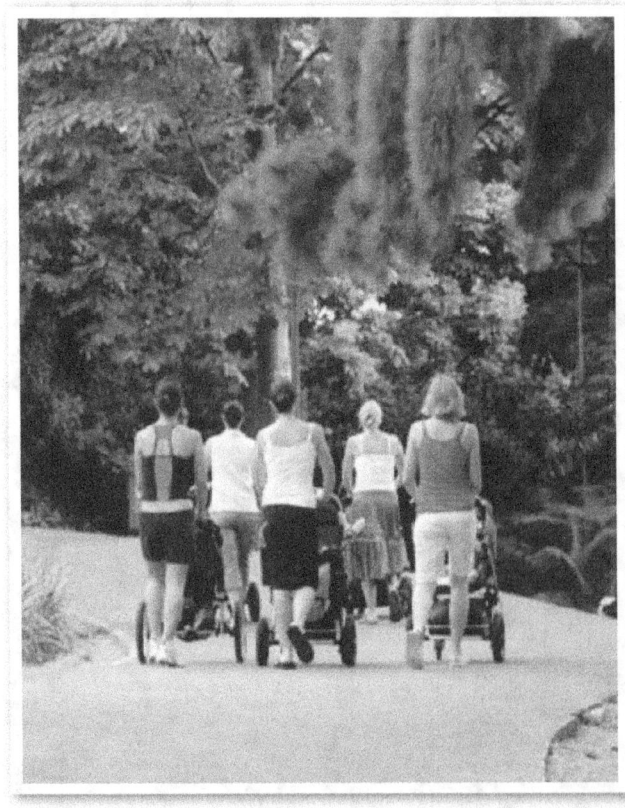

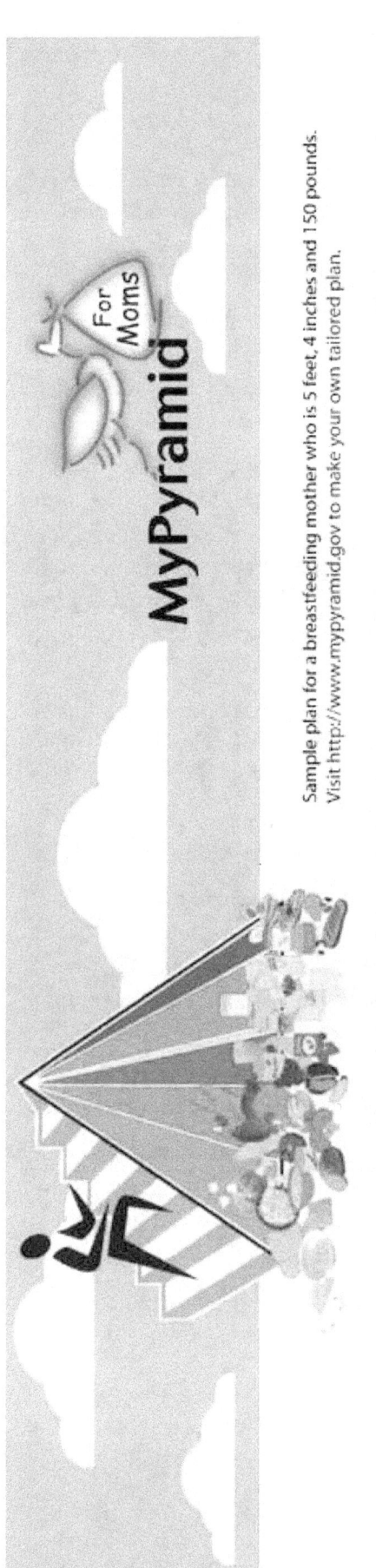

MyPyramid
For Moms

Sample plan for a breastfeeding mother who is 5 feet, 4 inches and 150 pounds.
Visit http://www.mypyramid.gov to make your own tailored plan.

	GRAINS Make half your grains whole	VEGETABLES Vary your veggies	FRUITS Focus on fruits	MILK Get your calcium-rich foods	MEAT & BEANS Choose lean with protein
Birth to 6 Months **Nov - May** Based on a 2400 calorie pattern*	**8 ounces a day** Aim for at least 4 ounces of whole grains a day	**3 cups a day** Aim for this much weekly: Dark green veggies - 3 cups Orange veggies - 2 cups Dry beans & peas - 3 cups Starchy veggies - 6 cups Other veggies - 7 cups	**2 cups a day** Eat a variety of fruit Go easy on fruit juices	**3 cups a day** Go low-fat or fat-free when you choose milk, yogurt, or cheese	**6½ ounces a day** Choose low-fat or lean meats and poultry. Vary your protein routine—choose more fish, beans, peas, nuts, and seeds.
6 to 12 Months **Jun - Nov** Based on a 2400 calorie pattern*	**8 ounces a day** Aim for at least 4 ounces of whole grains a day	**3 cups a day** Aim for this much weekly: Dark green veggies - 3 cups Orange veggies - 2 cups Dry beans & peas - 3 cups Starchy veggies - 6 cups Other veggies - 7 cups	**2 cups a day** Eat a variety of fruit Go easy on fruit juices	**3 cups a day** Go low-fat or fat-free when you choose milk, yogurt, or cheese	**6½ ounces a day** Choose low-fat or lean meats and poultry. Vary your protein routine—choose more fish, beans, peas, nuts, and seeds.

Know your limits on fats, sugars, and sodium

	OILS Aim for this much:	EXTRAS Limit extras (solid fats and sugars) to this much:
Birth to 6 Months	7 teaspoons a day	360 calories a day
6 to 12 Months	7 teaspoons a day	360 calories a day

* These are only estimates of your needs while you breastfeed. Check with your health care provider to make sure you are losing the weight gained during pregnancy.

The calories and amounts of food you need change over time while you are breastfeeding. Your Plan may show different amounts of food for different months, to meet your changing nutritional needs.

Handling Stress

Both short- and long-term stress can affect your body. In fact, stress can make you more likely to get sick. It can also make problems you already have worse. It can play a part in a range of issues, including trouble sleeping, stomach problems, headaches, and mental health conditions.

Having a new baby and learning how to breastfeed can be very stressful events. But it is important for mothers to take care of themselves. Try to listen to your body so that you can tell when stress is affecting your health, and take these steps to feel better!

- **Get help from a professional if you need it.** A therapist can help you work through stress and find better ways to deal with problems. For more serious stress-related disorders, like post-traumatic stress disorder, therapy can be helpful. There also are medications that can help ease symptoms of depression and anxiety and help promote sleep.

- **Relax.** It's important to unwind in a way that works for you. Try a bubble bath, deep breathing, yoga, meditation, and massage therapy. If you can't do these things, take a few minutes to sit, listen to soothing music, or read a book.

- **Sleep.** Your stress could get worse if you don't get enough sleep. It is hard to fight off illness when you sleep poorly. With enough sleep, it is easier to cope with challenges and stay healthy. Try to get seven to nine hours of sleep every night. If you can't, try to sleep when the baby sleeps.

- **Eat right.** Try to fuel up with fruits, vegetables, proteins, and whole grains. See **pages 39-41** for more nutrition information.

- **Get moving.** Physical activity not only helps relieve your tense muscles but helps your mood too! Your body makes certain chemicals, called endorphins, before and after you exercise. These relieve stress and improve your mood. If you are a new mother, ask your doctor when it is okay to start exercising.

- **Talk to friends.** Friends can be good listeners. Finding someone who will let you talk freely about your problems and feelings without judging you does a world of good. It also helps to hear a different point of view. Friends will remind you that you're not alone.

- **Compromise.** Sometimes, it's not always worth the stress to argue. Give in once in awhile.

- **Keep a journal.** Write down your thoughts. Have you ever typed an e-mail to a friend about your lousy day and felt better afterward? Why not grab a pen and paper and write down what's going on in your life! Keeping a journal can be a great way to get things off your chest and work through issues.

- **Help others.** Helping someone else can help you. Help your neighbor, or volunteer in your community.

- **Get a hobby.** Find something you enjoy. Make sure to give yourself time to explore your interests.

- **Set limits.** Figure out what you can really do. There are only so many hours in the day. Set limits with yourself and others. Don't be afraid to say no to requests for your time and energy.

- **Plan your time.** Think ahead about how you're going to spend your time. Write a to-do list. Figure out which tasks are the most important to do.

- **Don't deal with stress in unhealthy ways.** This includes drinking too much alcohol, using drugs, or smoking, all of which can harm the baby. It is also unhealthy to over-eat in response to stress.

Did You Know?

Breastfeeding can help mothers relax and handle stress better. Skin-to-skin contact with your baby has a soothing effect.

Questions to Ask Your Baby's Doctor

Use this tear-out form to write down questions you have for your baby's doctor and bring it to your next visit.

If your baby is not eating well or if you are concerned about your baby's health, call the pediatrician right away.

1. _____

_____

2. _____

_____

3. _____

_____

4. _____

_____

5. _____

_____

6. _____

_____

7. _____

_____

Questions to Ask Your Health Care Provider

Use this tear-out form to write down questions you have for your health care provider and bring it to your next visit.

If you have symptoms of an infection (see **page 21**) or urgent health concerns, call your health care provider right away.

1. _____

_____

2. _____

_____

3. _____

_____

4. _____

_____

5. _____

_____

6. _____

_____

7. _____

_____

Feeding Chart

Mark your baby's feedings in the chart below. The times should be when the feeding begins. You can note how long the baby fed at each breast. But keep in mind that feeding times will vary. Your baby will let you know when he or she is finished eating. If you are feeding pumped breast milk, include the amount your baby eats.

	Mon	Tue	Wed	Thurs	Fri	Sat	Sun
6 a.m.							
7 a.m.							
8 a.m.							
9 a.m.							
10 a.m.							
11 a.m.							
12 p.m.							
1 p.m.							
2 p.m.							
3 p.m.							
4 p.m.							
5 p.m.							
6 p.m.							
7 p.m.							
8 p.m.							
9 p.m.							
10 p.m.							
11 p.m.							
12 a.m.							
1 a.m.							
2 a.m.							
3 a.m.							
4 a.m.							
5 a.m.							

Diaper Tracker

You do not have to track diapers for a month to know your baby is eating well, but some women find it helpful to write it down. Weight gain is the best way to know if your baby is eating well. Talk to your baby's doctor if you are concerned.

Baby's Age	Number of Wet Diapers	Number of Bowel Movements	Color and Texture of Bowel Movements
Day 1 (first 24 hours after birth)			
Day 2			
Day 3			
Day 4			
Day 5			
Day 6			
Day 7			
Day 8			
Day 9			
Day 10			
Day 11			
Day 12			
Day 13			
Day 14			
Day 15			
Day 16			
Day 17			
Day 18			
Day 19			
Day 20			
Day 21			
Day 22			
Day 23			
Day 24			
Day 25			
Day 26			
Day 27			
Day 28			
Day 29			
Day 30			

Health Information from the Office on Women's Health

The Office on Women's Health (OWH) offers free women's health information on more than 800 topics through our toll-free call center and website, http://www.womenshealth.gov. Other information resources include:

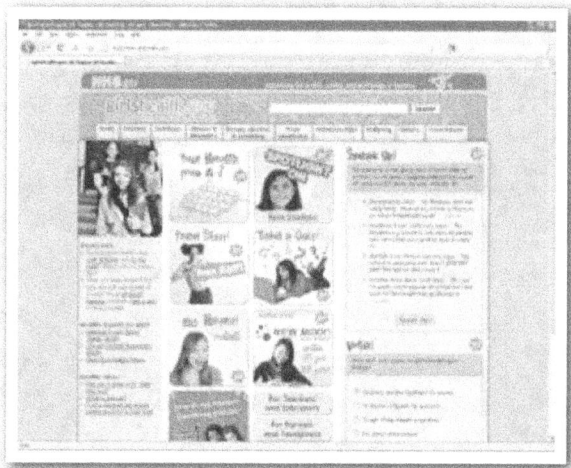

http://www.girlshealth.gov
Helping girls learn about health and growing up

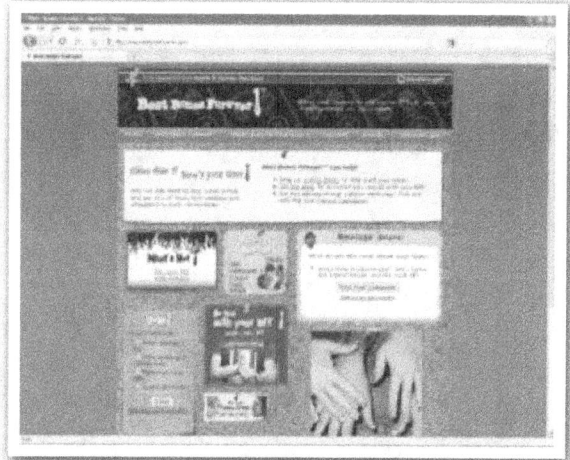

http://www.bestbonesforever.gov
Helping girls build strong bones

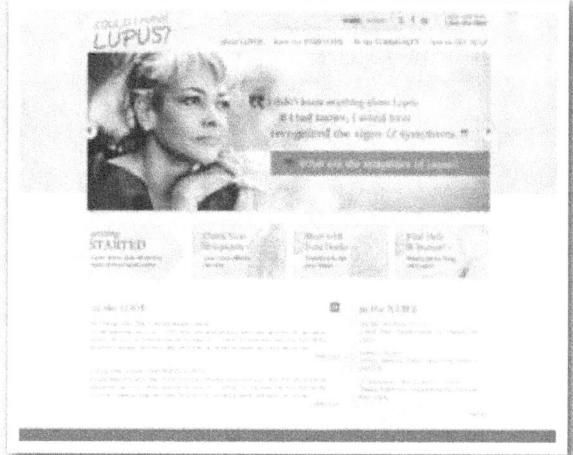

http://www.couldihavelupus.gov
Providing an online community for women with lupus

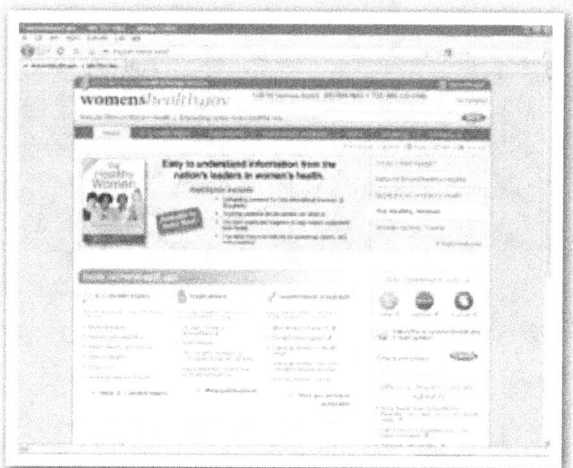

http://www.womenshealth.gov
Empowering women to live healthier lives